Contents

Introduction

YOU are probably reading this book because you or your child has asthma and you would like to know more about what asthma is, how to recognize it, and how best to treat it. You no doubt have many questions about asthma, such as: How do you recognize when you have asthma? Is it due to allergies? Can it be cured or effectively controlled? Is it due to emotional stresses? Will my child grow out of it? Could asthma be due to my occupation? You will find these and many more questions answered in this book.

The purpose of this book is to inform people with asthma or close to someone with asthma, about what is known today regarding this group of inflammatory* conditions of the airways, which lead to the episodes of shortness of breath, chest tightness, wheezing, and cough known as "asthma."

Although asthma has been recognized for more than 2,000 years and a variety of folk remedies used to treat it, it is only in the past 50 years that increasingly effective treatments have been developed and in the past 15 years that major strides have been made in understanding and controlling the condition. As a result, it is now possible to treat about 95 percent of all asthmatics so well that they should hardly know they have the disease and should be able to carry on normal, active lives at work and at play. **Unfortunately, these developments have not yet reached the majority of patients who might benefit from them**, and it may be partly for this reason that asthma seems to be getting more frequent and more severe. More people with the disease are being admitted to hospitals and, most unfortunately, the death rate from asthma, particularly in young and middle-aged people, has been increasing throughout the world. This increase has been quite striking in some countries and less obvious in others.

We have written this book because we think that the best way to combat the increasing death rate from asthma is to inform asthmatics about modern methods of investigation and treatment, in the hope that they will work closely with their doctors to ensure they receive the best available assessment and treatment.

Above all, since people with asthma should know almost as much about **their own** disease as their doctor, this book is intended to teach you, the person with asthma, to understand your disease so well that you can undertake self-care of it on a daily basis, determine when you are getting worse, and correct deterioration long before you require hospital treatment.

We hope that, with time, using the information in this book and with the confidence that comes from successfully taking care of your asthma, you will be unhampered by the unpredictability of poorly treated asthma and so be able to lead a healthy, happy life.

---

* As you will see in detail in *Chapter 5*, inflammation is a reaction of the lining of the airways to injury, which leads to narrowing of the air passages. It is this narrowing that leads to most of the obvious features of this condition.

Conquering Asthma

An Illustrated Guide to Understanding and Self Care for Adults and Children

PETER J. BARNES, MA, DM, DSc, FRCP

Professor of Thoracic Medicine
National Heart and Lung Institute
University of London
Honorary Consultant Physician
Royal Brompton Hospital, London, Great Britain

MICHAEL T. NEWHOUSE MD, MSc, FRCP(C), FRCP, FCCP

Clinical Professor of Medicine
McMaster University Faculty of Medicine
Director, Medical Aerosol Research Laboratory
St. Joseph's Hospital, Hamilton, Canada

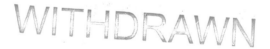

⊠ MANSON
PUBLISHING

Acknowledgments

We are particularly grateful for the joy of seeing Sari O'Sullivan use her considerable artistry to turn our vague concepts into beautiful illustrations, and we especially wish to thank Glaxo for permission to use many graphs and illustrations from their clinical teaching slide set.

Our grateful thanks are also due to the following for permission to use photographs or drawings: Simon Fraser/Science Photo Library (p. 10), Carlos Goldin/Science Photo Library (p. 10), OPCS/LAIA (p. 15), Ralph Hutchings (p. 17, 45, 118), Allen & Hanburys (p. 19, 20), Tom Daly (p. 19, 86, 91, 93, 101), Boehringer Ingelheim GmbH (p. 20), Dr Jennifer Sturgess (p. 21), Astra Draco/Dr Yelke (p. 25), Ann Dewar (p. 30), Janssen Pharma (p. 44), Hayward Medical Communications (p. 52), Heine Schneebeli/Science Photo Library (p. 119) and Alan Edwards (p. 134 × 3).

We should also like to thank our colleagues who, with the support of the Ontario Thoracic Society, produced the summary tables, Dr Christine Jenkins who made our text more applicable to readers in Australia and our secretaries Maureen McPhail, Janice Rutgers and Madeleine Wray for their assistance in preparing the manuscript.

Dedication

This book is dedicated to our patients from whom we have learned so much.

Peter J. Barnes
Michael T. Newhouse

Conquering Asthma — An Illustrated Guide to Understanding and Self Care for Adults and Children
ISBN: 1−874545−02−2

First published in Canada © 1991 by Decker Periodicals Inc, Hamilton, Ontario, under the International Copyright Union.

Revised and updated edition first published in Great Britain © 1994 by Manson Publishing Ltd, 73 Corringham Road, London NW11 7DL.

Colour reproduction by Tenon & Polert Ltd, Hong Kong
Typeset by Setrite Typesetters Ltd, Hong Kong
Printed and bound in Spain by Grafos SA, Barcelona

1   What Is Asthma?

THE chronic lung condition that doctors call asthma is not really a single disease, but rather a reaction of the air passages in the lungs to injury caused by a variety of agents.

Probably the most important thing to realize is that asthma is **inflammation** of the air passages. Injury to the air passages causes signals to be sent to the bone marrow to produce special cells such as eosinophils (see *Chapter 5*), which participate in the inflammation. It is as though the bone marrow is being told by the lining tissues of the air passages that they are being attacked by parasites. The defence set up by the body leads to inflammation, which causes swelling of the lining tissues of the air passages and "twitchiness" of the muscle layers in their walls. The result, if untreated, is ongoing narrowing of the air passages and episodes of muscle spasm that are the basis for the symptoms and signs of asthma.

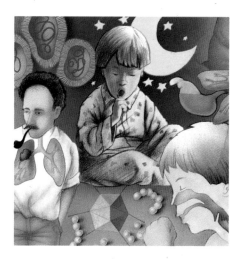

Inflammation, a characteristic of almost all asthma, is the underlying problem leading to all of the symptoms that you experience. It also causes the findings that your doctor notices when examining you, as well as the laboratory test findings that are seen with this condition. Understanding that this condition is a result of inflammation is also especially important because, in the past, doctors used to think that the problem was mainly one of narrowing of the airways, and so they treated asthma with relaxers of the airway muscle known as bronchodilators. These relaxers did not deal with the underlying problem, but simply **re-lieved** the **consequences** of the inflammation, namely constriction of the airways. Treating asthma in this way is a bit like treating appendicitis with pain killers **only**, while leaving the infected appendix in the body. In a similar way, if the inflammation that underlies asthma is treated only with bronchodilators, relief of the complaints is only temporary, and the underlying process smoulders on. This can lead to ongoing asthma attacks and sometimes permanent injury to the air passages, such as permanent narrowing.

It is clear then, that the underlying problem in asthma is **inflammation** and **not bronchoconstriction**, and the most effective approach to treating the disease is to treat the inflammation with continuing anti-inflammatory treatment (unless the asthma episodes are **very mild and infrequent**). This approach to treatment removes much of the need for bronchodilators (see *Chapter 10*).

I N recent years the media have been full of reports about asthma: about increases in how frequently this disease occurs in the population; about increases in severity of the disease, and particularly about considerable increases in death due to asthma. Naturally such reports are frightening to asthmatics and particularly to the parents of children with asthma. Apparent increases in asthma are blamed on the environment, especially in industrialized cities, on chemicals in the home and workplace, and on foods, particularly those that are processed and contain additives or preservatives.

THE HISTORY OF ASTHMA

Although these reports in the media suggest that asthma may be a new condition affecting mankind, asthma is actually a very old disease. As far as we know, asthma was first described in ancient Egypt over 3,500 years ago in the Ebers Papyrus. The condition was again mentioned about 2,500 years ago in the writings of the Greek physician Hippocrates, who named the disease *asthma*, which means gasping for breath or panting. Aretaeus, who lived during the reign of the Roman Emperor Trajan (A.D. 98–117), recognized that asthma was a chronic breathing condition that came and went spontaneously. He also recognized that asthma was related to exercise and first described the acute asthma attack. The first accurate description of the condition occurred during the late Roman Empire, when Galen (A.D. 130–200), court physician to the Roman Emperor Marcus Aurelius, wrote about it. Galen thought that asthma was related in some way to fluid pouring into the lungs from the brain. This idea probably arose from the fact that asthma is frequently associated with rhinitis and sinusitis, resulting in the discharge of secretions from the nose and a drip down the back of the throat (so-called "catarrh").

In the tenth century, Moses Maimonides, court physician to the Saracen general Saladin, Commander of the forces of Islam during the crusades, wrote of asthma that it was associated with sudden, unpredictable episodes of breathlessness and that it might improve during puberty. He suggested that chicken soup might be used to

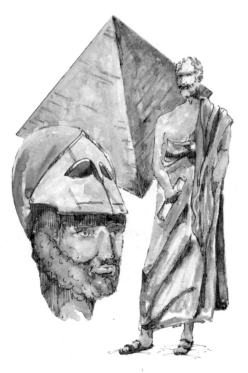

treat the condition! Subsequently, asthma was discussed by Paracelsus (A.D. 1493–1541), who argued against Galen's ideas that asthma might be due to a disturbance of the "humours" of the body. He thought that the illness was due to external causes.

Van Helmont, who lived in the early part of the seventeenth century and was himself an asthma sufferer, referred to the condition as "epilepsy of the lungs" because of the unpredictability, sudden onset, and severity of the attacks. He was probably also the first to recognize the association between the disease and contact with inhaled or ingested substances. He recognized that the condition might be inherited, and that it got worse under certain conditions of climate or emotional stress. Sir Thomas Willis and Thomas Sydenham, famous British physicians of the seventeenth century, both wrote of asthma, while the Italian physician Ramazzini was the first to clearly describe occupational asthma in bakers, grooms working with horses, and spinners or weavers exposed to flax, hemp, or silk.

The first book about asthma was written by Sir John Floyer towards the end of the seventeenth century. He was also an asthmatic who recognized the association of the disease with emotional stress, laughter, respiratory infections, and exercise. He first noted that asthma is often worse at night, based on his personal experience with frightening attacks that awoke him from sleep.

In the eighteenth century, Giovanni Morgagni, Professor of Anatomy in Padua, first described the thick secretions that had plugged the air passages of patients who died after a severe attack of asthma. He recognized that the condition could occur as a result of exposure to environmental factors such as hemp dust or feathers in bedding. At about the same time, John

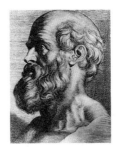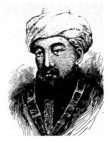

Hippocrates and Moses Maimonides.

Millar described the natural history of asthma in children and indicated that this condition was a definite disease separate from other diseases of the lung.

During the nineteenth century, when the scientific basis for medicine was being laid down by scientists like the great German pathologist Rudolph Virchow (1821–1902) and bacteriologists Louis Pasteur (1822–1895) and Robert Koch (1843–1910), aerosol therapy with extracts of the plant *Datura stramonium* (similar to the belladonna-derived compounds that we use today) were first described in the treatment of asthma. In 1819, the great French chest physician Laennec provided the first really accurate description of asthma and, by means of the stethoscope that he had developed, first noted the musical wheezing sounds that are so typical of the disease. He clearly distinguished asthma from other causes of breathlessness. At about the same time, it was recognized that attacks of asthma and hay fever often occurred together at the same time of year.

In 1864, Henry Hyde Salter, an English physician, wrote that the airways could be affected directly by a number of non-specific trigger factors that could cause paroxysms of asthma. These factors included exercise, cold air, laughter, coughing, and sneezing, as well as chemical and mechanical

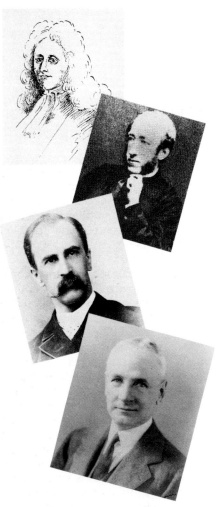

Sir John Floyer, Henry Hyde Salter, Sir William B Osler and Francis Rackemann.

the nose (rhinitis) and sometimes the lining of the eyelids (conjunctivitis) as well. It was also recognized that asthma could be allergic and caused by certain things in the environment such as pollens or animal danders. In addition, when the asthmatic condition was present, deterioration could occur quickly on increased exposure to the causative agents or when exposure occurred to certain "triggers," such as emotional stress, exertion, cold air, fog, or changes in the weather.

Because poorly controlled asthmatics tended to be anxious and depressed, Osler came to the unfortunate conclusion that asthma had a large "neurotic" component. This idea continued to hold considerable sway until fairly recently, when it was recognized that the so-called asthmatic personality is the result rather than the cause of the poorly controlled disease.

In the 1930s, it was suggested by the American allergist Rackemann that asthma could be divided into two types—one type was clearly due to some outside factor such as animal danders or pollens, while the other type somehow arose "from within" and was thought for a long time to be due to sensitivity to bacteria growing in the airway. The idea of bacterial hypersensitivity as a cause of asthma is no longer believed, and this so-called "intrinsic" asthma is now thought to be due perhaps to viral infection, although attempts to prove this have not yet been successful.

During the past twenty years, there have been rapid advances in our understanding of many of the fundamental mechanisms underlying asthma, but in spite of this, the cause of the disease remains elusive.

Skilled observations by these and other physicians have taught us that asthma is usually a chronic allergic illness that comes and goes sometimes

irritation. He also noted that asthma might occur as a result of exposure to grass and a variety of domestic and wild animals.

It became obvious to the outstanding physicians of the turn of the century, such as the German Hans Curshmann (1875–1950) and Canadian William Osler (1849–1919), who became Professor of Medicine at Oxford, that asthma was an inflammatory condition of the air passages in the lungs often associated with involvement of without an obvious cause, that while people often get very sick from it, particularly during infections such as viral chest colds, they rarely die of the disease, and that often the condition grumbles on for many years.

Nowadays we have better medications for treating this condition than ever before, and it is therefore doubly tragic that in many modern countries with excellent health care facilities, the asthma death rate remains unacceptably high and may even be rising. It is our hope that by the time you have

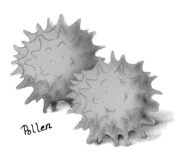

Pollen

finished reading this book, you will understand that most of these deaths are unnecessary and are occurring because available **preventative** measures to **control** asthma are not being used as often and as vigorously as they should be. During flare-ups of the disease, you the patient, frequently do not take the medications that will rescue you from an asthmatic attack soon enough or in adequate doses. This is because you do not have the necessary instructions and medications to keep on hand (and take with you when you are away from home on business or on holiday) or because you have not followed your doctor's instructions. Reducing the amount of illness and the death rate from asthma is a challenge to patients and their doctors. We have the medical tools — now let's get together and use them effectively to control asthma.

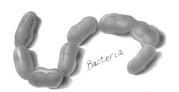

Bacteria

ASTHMA AND THE ENVIRONMENT

OUTDOOR POLLUTION

There has recently been considerable interest in whether environmental factors may be important in asthma. There has been particular concern about whether atmospheric pollution may be a factor contributing to the worsening of asthma.

There are several pollutants which are present in the atmosphere that are known to trigger wheezing or to make the airways more twitchy when given to patients with asthma. *Sulphur dioxide* (or SO_2) gas is an irritant gas that used to reach high levels in the atmosphere in cities with factories, but is now much less of a problem with the introduction of Clean Air legislation in many countries which has limited the amount of air pollution. Asthmatics develop wheezing and coughing when exposed to sulphur dioxide in the laboratory, since this gas is very irritant. However, the amount of sulphur dioxide needed to have this effect, even in patients with severe asthma, is never normally reached in the atmosphere.

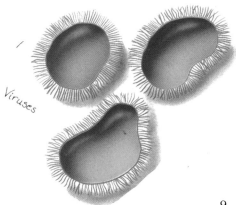

Viruses

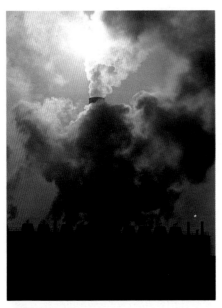

Industrial pollution — a power station in Bitterfeld, eastern Germany.

Another atmospheric pollutant is *nitrogen dioxide* (or NO_2) which may be found in car exhaust fumes and therefore is particularly found in inner cities and in the vicinity of motorways. Nitrogen dioxide has been shown to make the airways of asthmatics more twitchy, but again much higher concentrations are required than are normally found in the atmosphere.

Ozone, which is generated in the atmosphere by the action of sunlight, is found both in cities and in the countryside. The levels may be high in the smogs of cities such as Los Angeles and Athens, but may also be high in other areas under certain climatic conditions. Ozone may cause airway twitchiness both in normal and asthmatic individuals and laboratory studies have shown that ozone can even cause inflammation of the airways. However, the concentrations needed to produce these effects are much greater that the highest levels that occur in the atmosphere.

Dust particles may also cause irri-

tation of the airways and could lead to wheezing. Indeed it is probably the dust particles from coal burning fires and factories which were the main pollutant in the terrible smogs and fogs that used to occur in London in the 1950s.

Whether these pollutants are linked to asthma symptoms and attacks has recently been looked at in some detail. Several studies have attempted to relate the frequency of asthma symptoms or attacks to the levels of pollutants in the atmosphere. In general there is no convincing evidence that individual pollutants are associated with the worsening of asthma, either in terms of increasing symptoms such as wheezing, or in triggering more severe attacks. However, it is possible that there may be an interaction between different atmospheric pollutants, leading to greater effects on the airways than would be predicted from the studies with individual pollutants in isolation. It is also possible that pollutants may increase the re-

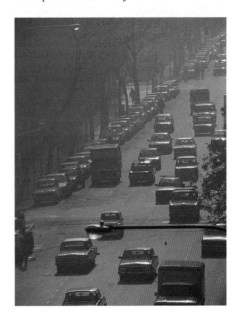

Smog in Buenos Aires, Argentina.

action to other factors, such as allergens in the atmosphere. For example, a recent study showed that exposing asthmatic patients to low concentrations of ozone that were themselves ineffective led to an increase in the response to an inhaled allergen. More research on this important topic is needed, particularly now that there is evidence of increasing air pollution from car exhaust and diesel fumes. There are several other substances from car exhausts, such as hydrocarbons, which may also have a deleterious effect on the airways, but they have not yet been studied in detail.

INDOOR POLLUTION

Perhaps the commonest form of indoor pollution is *cigarette smoking* and the effects of passive smoking (inhaling other people's cigarette smoke). It is common for patients with asthma to develop coughing, wheezing and chest tightness when they enter a room filled with cigarette smoke. Cigarette smoking can trigger asthma symptoms and few asthmatics smoke as a consequence. But what about passive smoking? There is some evidence that exposure to passive smoking may be associated with a greater likelihood of developing asthma in children and a greater risk of developing other allergic diseases (such as rhinitis and eczema). This may partly be due to the effects of smoking during pregnancy and there is now persuasive evidence that smoking during pregnancy is associated with an increased risk of the child developing a tendency to allergic diseases. Exposure to passive cigarette smoke during early childhood may also have some risk for developing asthma (particularly if the mother smokes), but there are very few studies that have looked into the relative risk of developing asthma with the amount of cigarette smoke inhaled in the home. The best advice that can be given is to avoid active and passive cigarette smoke exposure and parents of children with asthma must be discouraged from smoking especially at home.

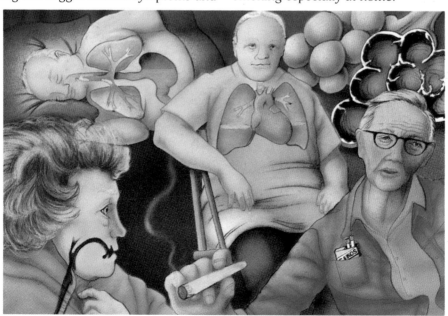

Smoking can damage your lungs and is certainly not recommended for asthmatics.

Another form of indoor pollution is exposure to *house dust mites*, particularly in the bedrooms. House dust mites flourish in warm humid conditions and like to live in air-conditioned rooms. The increase in central heating in bedrooms and the use of carpets in the bedroom favour the proliferation of house dust mites.

This could be one of the factors contributing to the increased problems with asthma in many countries.

Nitrogen dioxide may also be found in high levels in some homes especially where ventilation is poor, as it is given off by certain cookers and gas heaters and could be a factor in asthma symptoms.

3 How Common is Asthma?

THERE'S A LOT OF IT ABOUT

Asthma is one of the most common of all diseases. Although there are some variations in the number of asthmatics in different countries, most surveys have shown similar numbers of people affected, particularly when the same questions are used to find out whether or not someone has asthma. (Everyone who wheezes does not necessarily have asthma!) Of course there are difficulties working out how common asthma is in a population because symptoms come and go, and asthma is more common at certain ages (such as during childhood). In most industrialized countries, between 3 and 6 percent of the population — that is, one out of every 15 to 30 adults — have asthma. In childhood the figure rises to as high as one child in every five and is more common in boys than in girls, for reasons that are not understood.

IS ASTHMA BECOMING MORE COMMON?

Several recent surveys have suggested that asthma is becoming more common. This is against the trend for all other treatable conditions, and it makes asthma one of the few common treatable conditions in the world that is increasing. Surveys in Australia and New Zealand have shown that the number of children diagnosed with asthma has doubled over the last twenty years. The most likely explanation would be that we are better at diagnosing asthma today, but this has been taken into account in the surveys, so there must be other explanations. In a recent survey in England, it was found that twice as many people were going to see their doctors with asthma than 10 years ago. Other evidence also points towards an increased amount of asthma, and there is further evidence that asthma is becoming more troublesome and needs more treatment than previously. Thus, more people are having to go into hospital with asthma attacks, and there is some indication that many people are having more severe asthma attacks. Fortunately, very few asthmatic patients die from asthma, but recently there has been a trend for fatal asthma attacks to increase in several countries, particularly in New Zealand, where the increase in deaths from asthma has been especially noticeable. Although the cause of the increased deaths from

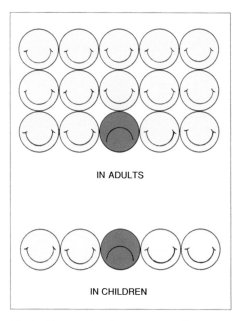

IN ADULTS

IN CHILDREN

The incidence of asthma among adults and children.

13

asthma is still in dispute, all the surveys seem to point to the fact that patients who die are **not receiving enough treatment** for their asthma — and certainly have not been taking enough "preventer" or anti-inflammatory treatments (see *Chapter 10*). Some doctors have suggested that overuse of "reliever" inhalers may account for some of the increased asthma deaths. Most evidence indicates that this is not true; rather, asthma deaths are usually due to too little treatment being started too late.

Why is there more asthma around? The reasons are not yet known. One possibility is that there are more allergic factors in the atmosphere. House dust mite, which is a very common allergic factor, thrives in warm rooms, and central heating may allow these mites to survive in large numbers in bedrooms, whereas previously they would struggle against the cold blasts of air from open windows. In some countries, an increase in pollen from trees and shrubs has led to increases

in asthma. In Kuwait and Arizona, USA, which have a dry, desert climate, asthma was almost unknown until the discovery of oil in the former and the development of retirement communities in the latter led to far greater prosperity. This allowed the planting of trees that could now be watered regularly. There was an enormous increase in hay fever and asthma, which was related to the increase in pollen grains in the air. Industrial pollutants may also contribute to the increase in asthma, and certain substances in car exhaust fumes have come under suspicion. Even diet may play its part — there is reason to think that increased consumption of animal fats might lead to greater inflammatory changes, since some inflammatory chemicals that may be involved in asthma are derived from these fats. Indeed, switching to a diet with less animal fat and more fish oil might improve asthma. Asthma is almost unknown among the Inuit of arctic Canada, who are exposed to little pollen and live on a diet of fish in

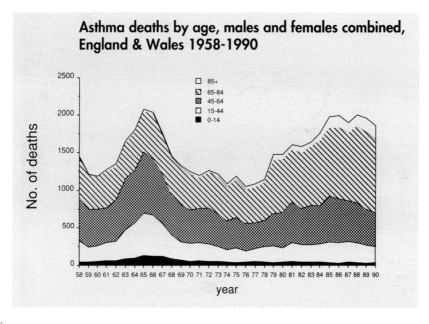

Asthma deaths by age, males and females combined, England & Wales 1958-1990

relatively isolated communities. There is also some evidence that increased salt intake may be associated with an increase in asthma. None of these theories has been proved, and more research needs to be done to find out just why asthma is on the increase, in sharp contrast to other treatable diseases.

ASTHMA — AN INTERNATIONAL DISEASE

Asthma occurs in every country in the world, although there may be sharp differences between different countries. Most industrialized countries have a similar amount of asthma, and the figures for the USA, Canada, UK, France, Germany, Australia, and New Zealand are about the same. In Japan, however, asthma appears to be somewhat less common. In some countries, like New Guinea, asthma was so rare that there was no native word for the disease, although recently there has been a steep rise in the amount of asthma there. In other parts of the world, asthma may be very common.

On the small, isolated island of Tristan da Cunha, in the South Atlantic, almost half of the population have asthma — this is because several of the original settlers had asthma and there has been interbreeding. This demonstrates the importance of inherited (genetic) factors in predisposing to some kinds of asthma, especially the allergic type.

Surveys of asthma in developing countries have demonstrated that asthma is more common in towns than in the countryside. For instance, in villages in Kenya, asthma is almost unknown, but is increasingly seen in the towns. In Australia, however, there is no significant difference in asthma prevalence for rural or urban communities. Why urbanization should lead to increased asthma is not yet known, as several factors may change — the standard of living may be higher, the diet may become more westernized (less roughage, more animal fats), and there may be fewer parasitic infestations. In westernized countries, such contrasts of asthma frequency are not found, as differences between village

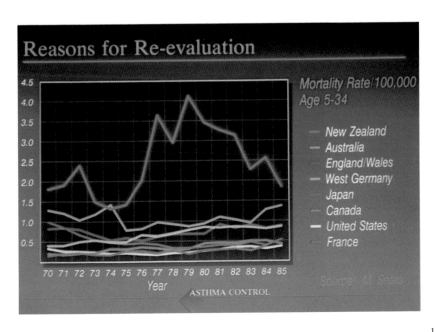

and town are not as marked. A striking example of asthma changing with the movement of a population is provided by the Tokelau islanders. The whole population of the small Tokelau Islands, in the South Pacific, was forced to move to New Zealand when the islands were hit by a hurricane. Asthma was uncommon in children on the Islands but became very common when they lived in New Zealand. Similarly, asthma is much less common in West Indian children living in the Caribbean than in West Indian children born in the UK. This suggests that, regardless of origin, the amount of asthma depends on the place where people live and that factors in the environment and surroundings determine the amount and severity of asthma.

4 How Our Lungs Work

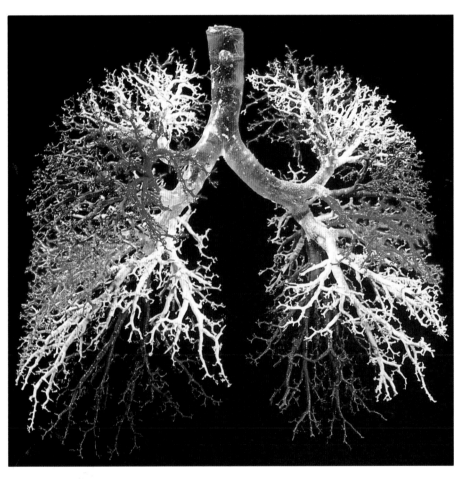

Cast of the bronchial tree.

THE NORMAL AIR PASSAGES AND LUNGS

Your lungs are two large, balloon-like structures inside the chest, one on each side of the heart, and they more or less completely fill the rib cage. The ribs and muscles of the chest wall protect the lungs from injury. Each lung is like a sponge and is made up of millions of tiny airspaces. These little air sacs (called *alveoli* after the Greek word for bunches of grapes) are lined by a thin, delicate, cellophane-like barrier between the air in the air sacs and a rich network of blood vessels that surrounds each sac. The total area of these air sacs would be as large as a tennis court if laid out flat. The whole structure of the lung is designed for efficient transfer of gas across this delicate membrane, and the large surface area allows for efficient exchange.

Oxygen from the air that is breathed in crosses into the blood vessels and then passes into the red blood corpuscles, which are pumped around the body in the bloodstream by the heart and supply oxygen to the various parts of the body. Oxygen is needed by all cells in the body to work normally because it enables the fuel (the food you eat) to be "burned."

The other function of the lung is to carry away the waste gas, carbon dioxide, that is formed as cells use foodstuffs and oxygen to provide the energy needed for your body to work properly. Carbon dioxide from the cells dissolves in the blood and, when it reaches the lungs, passes through the air sacs like the gas that fizzes out of a bottle of beer when it is opened. It is then expelled from your body when you breathe out.

Thus, the lung acts as an exchanger of gases: oxygen is passed in to be supplied for the needs of the body, whereas carbon dioxide is passed out. In order for this gas exchange to occur, it is necessary for air to get in and out of the lung. This is achieved by a series of branching tubes or airways. Air comes in from the mouth and across the voice box (*larynx*) into the main airway or windpipe (called the *trachea*). This divides into two airways (called *main bronchi*), which supply the left and right lung. The airways (or bronchi) then branch like a tree as the airways get smaller and smaller, until they are as thin as a piece of thread. The air sacs then branch like bunches of tiny grapes from these smallest airways.

Air passes through these airways from the mouth to the air sacs, where gas exchange takes place. The lungs expand like bellows to draw air in. Muscles in the chest (between the ribs) and the diaphragm, a muscle that forms a barrier between the lungs and the contents of the abdomen, expand the chest to create a slight vacuum so that air is drawn in through the airways. When these muscles relax, the lungs are allowed to retract, and air is pumped out again. Normally we breathe at about 10 to 12 breaths per minute, but under conditions where we need more oxygen, such as during exercise, we breathe faster and deeper. Sensors in the bloodstream and in the brain can detect the levels of oxygen and carbon dioxide and automatically regulate the rate and depth of breathing so that exactly the right amount of oxygen is supplied for the body's needs.

THE AIRWAYS

The airways, from the windpipe down to the smallest air passages that supply the air sacs, have a similar structure. They are lined by a delicate membrane. The cells right on the surface have very fine hairs (called *cilia*), (*see* page 20) which beat together in the same direction to waft the thin layer of phlegm or mucus that normally lines the airways towards the mouth. This

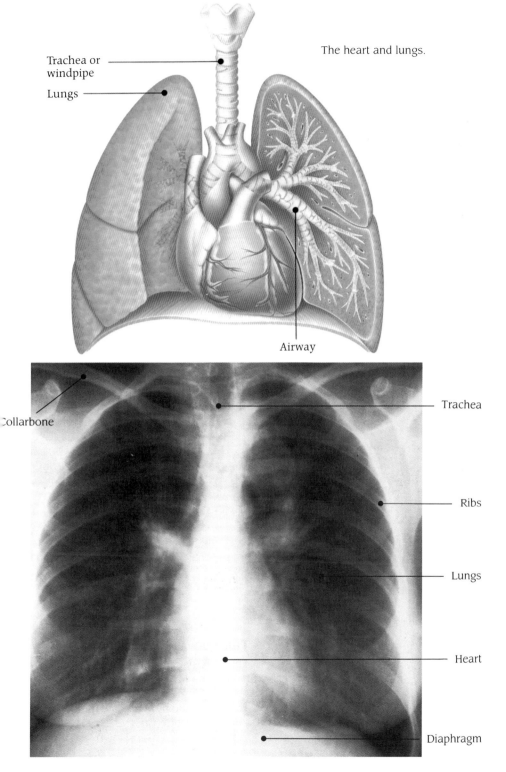

The heart and lungs.

Trachea or windpipe

Lungs

Airway

Collarbone

Trachea

Ribs

Lungs

Heart

Diaphragm

A chest x-ray.

mucus blanket traps dust particles that have been breathed in and stops them from reaching the air sacs. The mucus layer is formed by a mucus "factory" consisting of cells that are present in the lining membrane, and also by glands in the larger airways (*see* figure on page 21). These form most of the phlegm we cough up. The surface of the airways is always kept moist and a thin layer of fluid always coats the lining of the airway. If the surface should dry out, this may lead to problems in asthma.

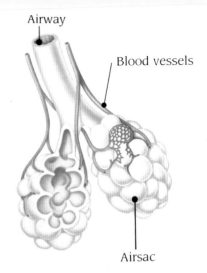

The airsacs and blood vessels.

Underneath the airway lining is a layer of muscle. If this muscle constricts, it leads to narrowing of the airway as the tube becomes squeezed. This muscle layer goes from the windpipe right down to the smallest airways. The true purpose of this muscle, which is not under voluntary control, is not really understood. Perhaps its original purpose was to suddenly narrow the airways to prevent large particles from entering the depths of the lung, or possibly it serves to strengthen the airways to prevent them from collapsing when air is sucked in. Whatever the function of the airway muscle normally, it certainly plays a very important role in asthma, as discussed in the next chapter.

Between the muscle layer and the delicate lining layer lies spongy tissue that has a rich blood supply. The larger airways (the bronchi) are strengthened by a tough, gristly structure called *cartilage*, which is in the form of rings around the largest airways. The windpipe appears corrugated because of the bands of cartilage. Since the cartilage is tough, it forms a kind of skeleton or scaffold that supports the large main airways and prevents them from collapsing when the vacuum action of the lung sucks air into the air sacs under negative pressure. The smallest air-

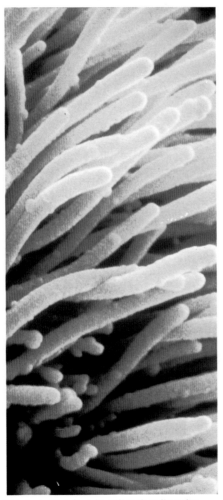

The hair-like fronds (cilia) that line the airways.

Cross-section of the airways.

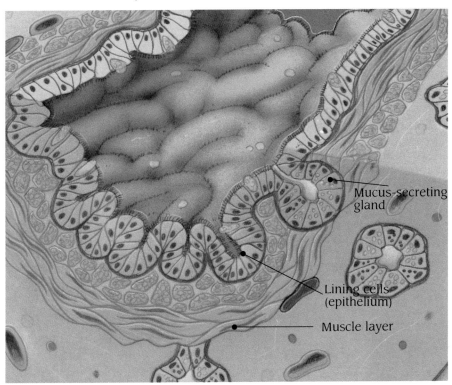

Mucus-secreting gland

Lining cells (epithelium)

Muscle layer

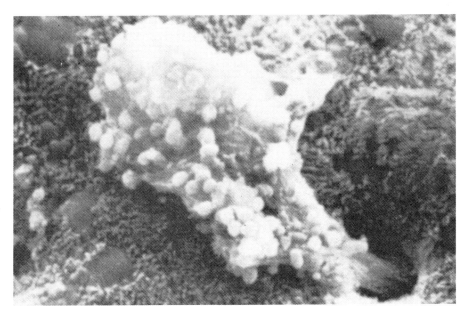

Mucus-secreting gland.

ways do not have this cartilage, but are normally held open mainly by the pull of the elastic tissues in the sponge-like lung substance. Because of this, the small airways are more likely to close off in an asthma attack.

THE NOSE

The nose also forms part of the airway system. Normally, people breathe through the nose, which acts as a filter to the air breathed in, and any large particles are trapped in the nose. The nose also acts as a natural air conditioner and warms and humidifies the air as it passes through on its way into the lungs. The nose has a delicate lining, like the airways, but when you get a cold (which may be due to a number of different viruses) or in an allergic reaction (such as breathing in pollen grains if you are allergic to pollens), the lining of the nose swells up (leading to blockage) and forms watery secretions (runny nose). Irritation of the nerves in the lining of the nose may cause sneezing. People who have asthma commonly also have this allergic reaction in the nose, which is called *rhinitis*, or hay fever if it occurs in the pollen season.

Now that we have reviewed the structure of the normal lung and airways and discussed their functions, it is possible to understand what goes wrong in asthma.

How Damage to the Air Passages Can Lead to Asthma

RECENTLY there have been important steps forward in finding out the underlying causes of asthma. Our improved understanding of asthma comes from research done in universities and by pharmaceutical companies. This research is the key to our understanding of how asthma should be treated.

"TWITCHY TUBES"

When you get sunburn, your skin becomes extremely sensitive to any additional injury. This is because the skin becomes inflamed by the sun's burning rays. Similarly, one of the features of asthma is the increased sensitivity or "twitchiness" of the airways. Asthmatic airways have greatly increased sensitivity to dusts, fumes, and certain

Cross-section of a blocked airway.

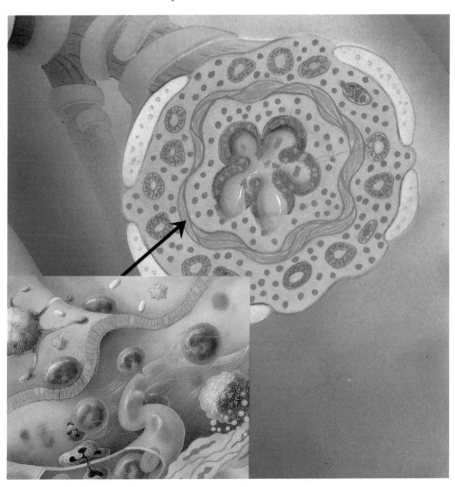

chemicals that are breathed into the lungs, compared to normal airways. For instance, cigarette smoke may have little effect when breathed in by normal people, but may cause coughing and wheezing in asthmatics. Similarly, breathing in cold air may trigger wheezing in the asthmatic patient, but has no effect in normal individuals. The phenomenon of increased twitchiness is fundamental to understanding asthma, as the degree of twitchiness is closely related to the severity of the asthmatic condition. Thus, the more twitchy the airways become, the more pronounced the wheezing and shortness of breath, particularly wheezing at night, and the more treatment is needed to control the symptoms. How airway irritability is measured is described in *Chapter 9*.

INFLAMMATION

Many years ago it was noticed that the lungs of asthmatic patients who died of a severe attack showed signs of marked inflammation in the airways. What is inflammation? Inflammation is the response the body makes to injury by various agents such as excessive heat, cold, radiation, chemicals, bacteria, or parasites. It consists of a series of events following the injury that involves the injured cells, additional cells that come from the blood, and other local tissue cells. Just as your skin swells with a bad burn, in asthma, fluid leaks from the blood into the airway tissue following injury, causing swelling and engorgement of the tissues lining the air passages. The cells that come in (white blood cells) are specialized in attacking and killing invading germs. An example of inflammation is an infection of the skin, such as occurs with a cut that becomes infected. The skin becomes hot, red, and swollen, and is very sensitive to the touch. If examined under a microscope, many white blood cells are

seen, which gather at the site of injury and eventually form pus. This inflammatory reaction is nature's way of warding off infection and prevents infection from spreading into the bloodstream. Eventually the whole process usually settles down and the area heals. This inflammation is usually a beneficial reaction that defends us from attack. Inflammation is a double-edged sword, however, and can be harmful if turned on excessively or inappropriately. This is what seems to happen in asthma.

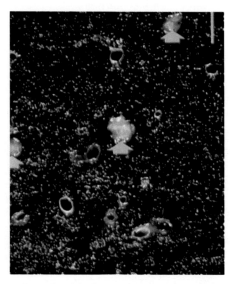

Mucus plug blocking airway. Arrows show the cut surface of the lung.

Recent research has shown that even the mildest of asthmatics have inflammation in the airways. In studies of asthmatic volunteers, tiny pieces of the airway lining have been collected through a telescope device, called a bronchoscope. In this way, it has been shown that, even in asthmatics who do not need any regular treatment, there are white cells in the lining of the airway, there are signs of swelling and leakage of blood, and most characteristically, the delicate layer of cells

24

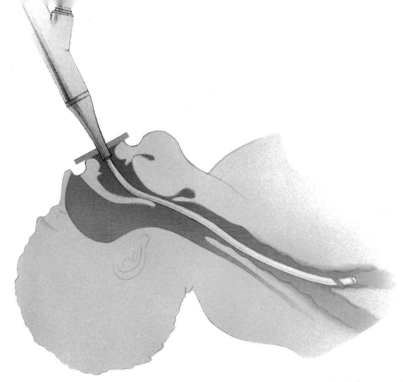

Bronchoscopy (top), and what the bronchoscope reveals (bottom): on the left, normal lungs; on the right, inflamed asthmatic lungs.

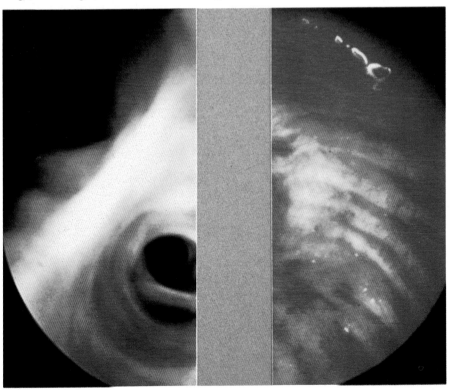

lining the airway may be damaged or shed. These findings are confirmed by other studies in which fluid has been washed into and out of the lungs through a bronchoscope. The fluid recovered has increased numbers of inflammatory cells. Furthermore, when asthmatic volunteers are exposed to allergic factors such as house dust mite or grass pollen, it can be shown that there is an increase in the inflammatory cells in the lung washings. The washings also have an increase in the amount of proteins derived from blood, giving evidence of leakage of blood vessels in the airways. This fits in with previous studies that have found an increase in these same proteins in the phlegm of asthmatics. Increased production of phlegm is seen in asthmatics and is also a feature of inflammation. The phlegm in asthma is very sticky and difficult to cough up. In severe asthma, it can completely block some of the smaller airways, which reduces oxygen getting to the air sacs and across into the bloodstream. Inflammation occurs in many other lung conditions, such as pneumonia (where it is helpful in warding off the infection) and in chronic bronchitis. But the inflammation that occurs in asthma is rather special. It differs from other inflammatory conditions because of the presence of a certain cell called the **eosinophil**.

EOSINOPHIL — FRIEND OR FOE?

Eosinophils are a specialized type of white blood cell. Their name is derived from the fact that they stain with a red dye called eosin, so they can be easily recognized when seen under a microscope. Eosinophils are known to be involved in worm and parasite infections and are part of the body's defence against these infections. Eosinophils contain nasty substances for example, a chemical called major basic protein that help to kill worms and parasites.

At one time it was thought that eosinophils were helpful in asthma and that they mopped up some of the chemicals that contribute to the disease. It is now believed that they may play a crucial role in asthma, for the following reasons: First, eosinophils are found in the airways of nearly all asthmatics, even those people who need only infrequent treatment. Increased numbers of eosinophils are also found in the bloodstream of many asthmatics, and in their phlegm. Sometimes eosinophils are so numerous that they color the phlegm yellow or green, and doctors may interpret this as meaning infection. That is why many asthmatics are treated with antibiotics over and over again before the asthma is recognized as such and treated appropriately. The number of eosinophils in lung washes and in the bloodstream of asthmatics is closely related to the severity of the infection and to how twitchy the airways of asthmatics are.

But how could eosinophils help to produce the condition we call asthma? It has been shown that the chemicals they contain, as well as killing parasites, may also damage the lining of the airways, and that these chemicals are found at the places where the lining cells have been shed. Damage to these protective lining cells may then expose nerve endings and make them more likely to be triggered. The loss of these lining cells takes away factors that may protect the muscle from going into spasm.

CHEMICAL MEDIATORS

Cells that are called forth by inflammation can produce several chemicals that are thought to contribute to the features of asthma. Perhaps the best known of these chemicals is histamine, which is produced by a certain allergic cell (mast cell). Histamine causes spasm of airway muscle and also swelling of the airway lining, and

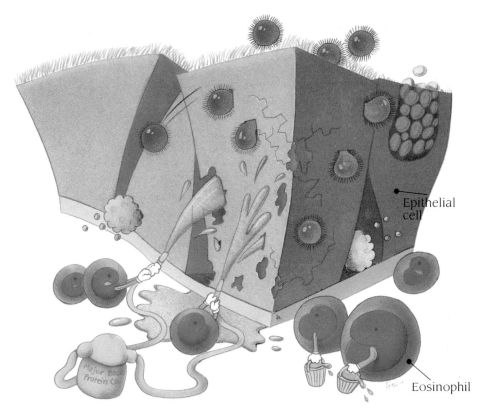

Epithelial cell

Eosinophil

Eosinophils enter the airways of asthmatic patients and release chemicals which damage the airway lining cells (epithelial cells).

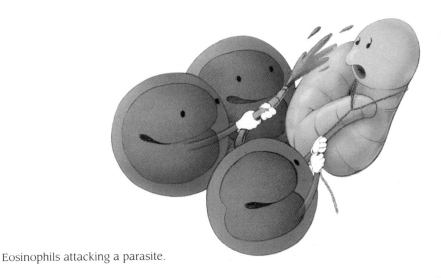

Eosinophils attacking a parasite.

so may be important in asthma. But antihistamines, which block the effects of histamine, are not very useful in treating asthma. That is because several other chemicals are also involved, and it would therefore be necessary to take a blocking medicine for each one. Thus, a whole pot full of pills, one for each chemical mediator, might be needed. One chemical that has attracted particular scientific interest recently is called platelet-activating factor, or PAF. When given to healthy people, PAF is able to mimic many of the characteristic features of asthma, including the airway twitchiness. Perhaps this is because PAF attracts eosinophils into airways and switches them on. It is interesting that two ancient Chinese herbal remedies for asthma, one from the leaves of the ginkgo tree and the other from a herb called hai-fen-teng, both contain PAF blockers. Folk remedies often contain some active chemical.

AIRWAY MUSCLE

Muscle spasm is an important part of asthma. The muscle that surrounds the airways is not under voluntary control, but goes into spasm in asthma. Several of the chemicals that may be involved in asthma can cause this spasm, as well as activation of certain nerves. When the muscle goes into spasm, this causes a narrowing of the airway so that air cannot easily pass in and out. This produces the wheezing sound that is so typical of asthma. Bronchodilator drugs may reverse this spasm and so usually relieve the wheezing and shortness of breath. It is important to realize that narrowing of the airways may also be due to swelling of the airway lining, and this narrowing is not relieved by bronchodilators to the same extent as muscle spasm. This may explain why your bronchodilator inhaler does not always work very well—particularly

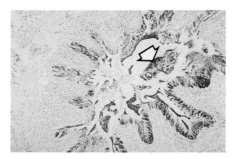

Cross-section of an airway from an asthmatic patient showing damage to the epithelium. The arrow is pointing to a clump of cells shed from the surface of the airway.

during a bad attack and why, at those times, much larger doses of the bronchodilator drugs may be needed.

NERVES

Many people believe that asthma is due to "nerves," meaning anxiety and stress. Although stress can trigger an asthma attack, just as exercise can, it is not the **cause** of asthma, as will be discussed in *Chapter 8*. Nerves in the other sense are the electrical wiring system of the body, sending messages rapidly from one part to another. Airways also have nerves in their walls. There are several types of nerves: some of them, for instance, lead to excessive muscle contraction or spasm, whereas others open the airways, that is, bronchodilate. Because of these opposing effects, it was thought that there might be some imbalance between the bronchoconstrictor and bronchodilator nerve systems, contributing to the twitchiness of the airway in asthma. There seems to be some truth in this theory. Of particular interest are the nerve endings close to the surface of the airway that can be triggered in asthma. These nerve endings may become exposed when the lining cells are damaged in asthma. Certain chemicals that are likely to be found in the inflammatory response can sensitize and trigger

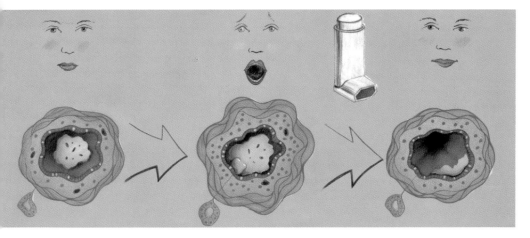

An airway constricts during an asthma attack. These constrictions are relieved by bronchodilator drugs.

these nerve endings, rather like the pain due to putting alcohol on a cut. Triggering of these nerve endings may cause coughing, which is common in asthma, and may cause symptoms of discomfort in the chest. Another symptom that some allergic asthmatics notice is an itching or tickling under the chin, which is also due to these nerve endings being triggered. As well as producing these symptoms of asthma, the triggering of these sensitive nerve endings may lead to bronchospasm through a reflex nervous pathway that travels via the spinal cord and may exaggerate the inflammatory response by causing more leakage and more production of phlegm.

ALLERGY AND ASTHMA

But what starts the whole process of asthma? The answer is not yet known, but in many asthmatics it is related to allergy.

What does allergy mean? Allergy is an excessive sensitivity to certain natural substances either in the atmosphere (e.g., house dust or pollen grains) or in food (e.g., shellfish or nuts) or to substances in the workplace. Allergy is an overreaction of the body's immune system, involving the excess production of certain proteins by the body (called antibodies), which react against the foreign substance. It is the tendency to overproduce these proteins that makes allergic people different from non-allergic people. Allergy can be shown by skin tests in which minute amounts of the foreign material, such as grass pollen, are injected into the skin (see Chapter 9). In people allergic to grass pollen, an itchy blister surrounded by an area of redness develops — this is the allergic response. About one in three people show such an allergic reaction in the skin to a few of the test substances (called allergens) when a whole battery of these substances are tested — so allergy is extremely common. It may affect people differently, sometimes as hay fever, sometimes as eczema, and sometimes as asthma. Of course, some of these conditions can occur together.

Scientists have discovered a lot about how allergy occurs. There are certain cells called mast cells. The name is derived from the German word "mast," which means "stuffed," since the cells are stuffed full of little packets that contain chemicals such as histamine. These cells are found close to

29

the surface of airways and sometimes actually within the airway. In allergic people, the surface of these cells may be coated with the allergic antibody. When a foreign protein, such as pollen grains, is breathed in, this reacts with the allergic protein and triggers the cells to release chemicals such as histamine. Histamine, as we have already discussed, can cause broncho-spasm, and this explains why breathing in something to which a person is allergic may also trigger an asthma attack. At one time it was believed that mast cells therefore held the key to understanding asthma, but we now know that they are only part of the story and that other allergic cells are also involved, particularly in the more prolonged episodes of wheezing.

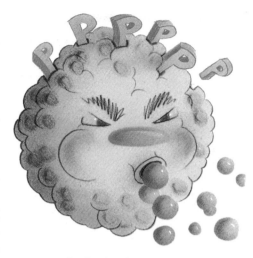

A mast cell releasing histamine.

(Below) Pollen cells—a greatly enlarged view, through the electron microscope.

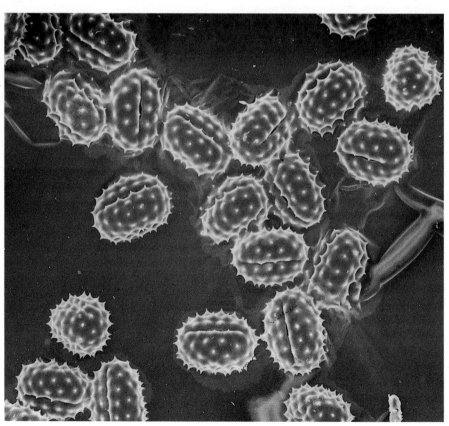

6 How to Tell if You or Your Child Have Asthma

WHEN asthma is absolutely typical, it is fairly easy to tell if you or your child has it, and this is especially true in older children and young adults. But in infants and younger children and in the late middle-aged and elderly, it can be much more difficult to be sure that it is really asthma that is causing the problem. This is because other conditions with similar features, but having a different cause and requiring different treatment, may be present. The conditions that may mimic asthma, thus confusing you and your doctor, will be discussed in *Chapter 7*.

ASTHMA: SOMETIMES A DIFFICULT DIAGNOSIS

Recent scientific studies have shown that asthma is not diagnosed as often as it should be, especially in children and the elderly. It is often called something else, such as croup or wheezy bronchitis in children and chronic bronchitis, emphysema, or heart failure in older age groups. This leads to incorrect treatment. Asthma may be difficult to diagnose because the lung and its air passages can only react to injury, no matter what the cause, in a limited number of ways. Thus, the features considered "typical" of asthma, such as breathlessness, wheezing,

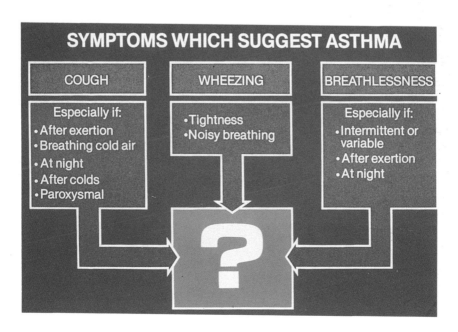

SYMPTOMS WHICH SUGGEST ASTHMA

COUGH	WHEEZING	BREATHLESSNESS
Especially if: • After exertion • Breathing cold air • At night • After colds • Paroxysmal	• Tightness • Noisy breathing	Especially if: • Intermittent or variable • After exertion • At night

chest tightness, and cough with phlegm production, may also occur in some people with other conditions, such as chronic bronchitis (most commonly related to many years of cigarette smoking) or heart disease with heart failure. Furthermore, in some asthmatics, especially small children, cough, particularly at night, may be the main feature of the condition, and wheezing may be rare or absent.

AIRWAY INFLAMMATION NARROWS AIR PASSAGES

The problems that you have because of asthma are the direct result of the injury to the airways resulting from contact with substances to which you may be allergic (such as pollens, animals, or dust), or a number of highly reactive chemicals that you may contact in your job (see *Chapter 15*), or factors as yet almost totally unknown (usually related to infection that, at first, looks like a bad chest cold perhaps caused by viruses or other virus-like agents). The most important thing to recall is that asthma is basically inflammation of the airways (see *Chapter 5*).

The features of hay fever with which many people are familiar are an example of inflammation of the lining of the nose. The changes inside the nose with hay fever are very much like those in the lining of the air passages of the lungs in asthma. In hay fever, which results from allergy to the pollen of the ragweed plant, the nasal passages become swollen and irritated, and there is overproduction of secretions. The result is obstruction of the passages, which, like the air passages of the lungs in asthma, become extremely sensitive to a variety of irritants such as cigarette smoke, car exhausts, perfumes, etc., leading to sneezing and running of the nose.

In ongoing or chronic asthma, the inflammation and its effects are present much of the time, but usually the severity varies a lot, so that the symptoms may vary considerably over short periods of time, within a few hours, from day to day, or from week to week. Alternatively, asthma may only be present during, and for a few weeks after, the pollen season. The features of asthma may, at first, come and go with varying periods of hours to days in between when you feel almost completely normal. With time and increasing severity, the asthma complaints may be present more and more of the time, and the relatively complaint-free periods between may be shorter and shorter. The very marked and spontaneous variability in complaints as well as the very noticeable improvement following treatment (see *Chapter 11*) with medications known as bronchodilators (*"relievers"*: drugs that open up airways by relaxing the smooth muscle lining the airway walls) or steroids (*"preventers"*: drugs that open up airways by reducing the inflammatory swelling and decreasing the secretions) are among the most important characteristics of asthma.

Now that you understand how the airways respond to injury, you will realize that you most likely have asthma if you experience episodes of shortness of breath and wheezing, often accompanied by chest tightness and cough. Sometimes with the cough there is sticky white or yellow phlegm, but often the cough is dry.

NOSE SYMPTOMS IN ASTHMA

Asthmatic episodes may be accompanied by nasal complaints or may be preceded for many months or even years by nasal problems such as runny nose, congestion due to secretions, and obstruction to the nasal passages due to swelling. When fairly mild, these episodes may appear like recurring colds that go to the chest, but differ from simple viral colds with cough because they seem to recur

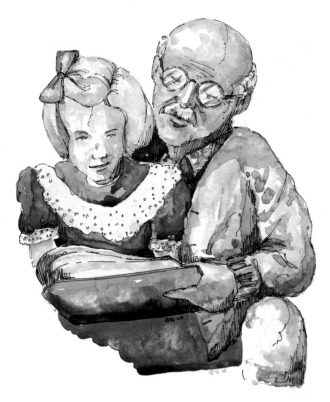

every few weeks and usually drag on for much longer than the normal 10 days or so expected of a viral illness affecting the nose and air passages of the lungs. Such nasal problems may precede the development of asthma by many years. Sometimes large swellings of the lining of the nose called *polyps* may completely plug the nasal passages, and these may need to be removed surgically on one or more occasions if they do not respond well to medical treatment.

NIGHT TIME SYMPTOMS

When asthma is poorly controlled and during flare-ups of asthma, symptoms tend to be worse at night, when they may seriously interfere with sleep (usually between 3:00 and 5:00 A.M.). On getting up in the morning, there is often a tight constricting feeling in the chest and increased cough, which is usually relieved temporarily by a bronchodilator (reliever) inhaler.

EXERCISE

Asthma attacks from exercise are typical of this condition and indicate that the disease is not well controlled (see *Chapter 8*).

FEATURES OF ASTHMA IN CHILDREN

In infants and very young children, it may be much more difficult to determine that they have asthma because the symptoms are often hard to distinguish from the typical chest infections commonly seen in childhood. Doctors sometimes call this condition "wheezy bronchitis" or, occasionally, croup. In this age group, asthma should be suspected if recurrent and persistent colds with cough (with or without wheezing) seem to follow rapidly one after the other and appear to drag on for several weeks.

During the episodic flare-ups, your child often wakes up repeatedly at night, and may keep the whole family awake with persistent coughing that may lead to retching and vomiting. The child sleeps restlessly and, being sleep deprived, often seems to be irritable all day as well. In the daytime, running and playing may lead to severe coughing spells. In kindergarten or school age children, the teacher will often send the child home repeatedly before the condition is recognized as asthma and properly treated because the constant coughing may disrupt the class. Thus, children with asthma may miss a lot of school (on average, 20 days or more per year), fall behind in their schoolwork, and develop behavioural problems.

Typically at first, family doctors or paediatricians try repeated courses of antibiotics, which do not appear to influence the condition much, if at all. In this age group, such complaints should make you suspect that asthma may be causing your child's problem and should lead to a thorough assessment by your family doctor, paediatrician, or by a lung specialist if your doctor thinks it necessary. A trial of adequate asthma treatment for several weeks or months will help you to see whether this will "break" the previous pattern of recurring illness and restore your child to normal health. The impression that asthma and not recurring infection is at the root of the problem is confirmed if attempts to gradually withdraw the asthma treatment lead to similar flare-ups.

In the allergic form of asthma, children often have eczema (an itchy, scaly rash mainly in skin creases in front of the elbows and behind the knee caps) for some time before the symptoms of asthma develop. Itchy red eyes (conjunctivitis) and nose symptoms (rhinitis) may also be present.

ASTHMA IN THE ELDERLY

The diagnosis of asthma in the elderly may also be difficult because heart disease, which requires totally different treatment, can sometimes imitate asthma. That is why, for many years, doctors labelled asthma-like complaints associated with heart failure, "cardiac asthma" (see *Chapter 7*).

PINPOINTING ASTHMA SOURCES

While the basic **cause** of inflammation of the air passages in asthma is still poorly understood, it is very important to try to relate the complaints to locations such as your home or workplace (see *Chapter 16*) or to exposure to a variety of domestic pets, particularly cats, dogs, hamsters, mice, or birds, foods (rarely), domestic animals, or to certain seasons of the year (e.g., pollens from spring until autumn or house dust during winter).

THE SEASONS AND ASTHMA

Complaints that commonly occur in spring are likely to be due to tree pollens, while complaints in the summer may be related to grass pollens (eg perennial rye grass), and those in the autumn to ragweed in some countries (USA, Canada) or to moulds. Particularly in cold climates, increased winter complaints may relate to house dust containing mites or household pets because houses are sealed up, thus concentrating the substances to which you may be allergic (*allergens*), while hot air heating systems spread the allergens around. Furthermore, cold air exposure during the winter months or occupations that expose workers to refrigeration may cause asthma flare-ups at the time of exposure.

In Australia and New Zealand because of the temperate climate, the house dust mite breeds all year round, although in late spring and late summer mite populations increase.

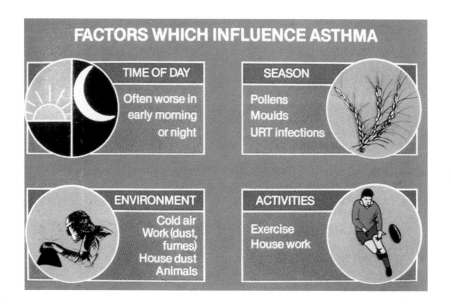

FACTORS WHICH INFLUENCE ASTHMA

TIME OF DAY
Often worse in
early morning
or night

SEASON
Pollens
Moulds
URT infections

ENVIRONMENT
Cold air
Work (dust,
fumes)
House dust
Animals

ACTIVITIES
Exercise
House work

FOOD AND DRUG ALLERGIES

Sometimes food allergies should also be considered. Foods commonly at fault include, among others, nuts (e.g., peanuts, Brazil nuts) and shellfish (shrimps, oysters), which may in a few asthmatics produce devastating attacks of asthma and swelling of the back of the throat, shutting off the windpipe. This overwhelming attack is called *anaphylaxis*. There may be associated collapse and shock. Severe and sudden asthma attacks may also occur, in a small proportion of asthmatics, a few minutes after taking aspirin or indomethacin and other similar drugs long used in the treatment of arthritis (see *Chapter 8*). Similar reactions may occur after eating foods preserved with the common food preservative sodium metabisulphite or very rarely from foods coloured with the yellow dye called tartrazine. Monosodium glutamate (MSG) added as a flavouring to Chinese food, in particular, may trigger so-called "chinese restaurant asthma" (see *Chapter 20* for more detail).

ASTHMA RELATED TO YOUR JOB

The workplace may also be the source of asthma symptoms, and this will be discussed in detail in another chapter (see *Chapter 16*). In trying to find the cause of your asthma, you should consider your job as a possible source of the difficulty. However, it may be difficult to sort this out because job-related asthma typically occurs not only during the day while you are actually on the job, but symptoms also occur and indeed are likely to be even more severe after you have been exposed all day and have returned home. This is because the inflammation that causes the complaints is the result of the exposure from many hours at work, and may reach its peak only several hours later when you are at home and perhaps asleep (doctors call this the "late reaction").

It is highly likely that your asthma is job-related if the asthma symptoms seem to get worse as the work week progresses, if there is improvement to some degree over the weekend, and if there is a great deal of improvement or even complete clearing while you are on a long holiday, only to have the symptoms return with gradually increasing severity after you go back to work. Occupations commonly associated with asthma and the mechanisms accounting for the problem are discussed in *Chapter 16.*

WHAT YOU TELL YOUR DOCTOR AT THE FIRST VISIT

The information that you give to your doctor (known as the history of the illness) is by far the most useful aid in sorting out the cause of any disease. This is certainly true of asthma where, as often happens, there may be no signs of the disease at all when you actually see your doctor. Even the simple test for airway narrowing performed by the doctor may show normality at that particular time. The lack of objective information at the time you see your doctor (especially if the account of the illness is not typical) sometimes leads to the incorrect idea that the episodes are due to "nerves." As a result, for nearly 100 years, doctors thought that asthma was a "neurotic" illness. This is definitely **not** true!

When you first go for medical attention, your doctor will ask you many questions and usually makes measurements of airway narrowing, namely measurements of peak expiratory flow, or performs a simple breathing test called *spirometry* (see *Chapter 9*). After bronchodilator inhalation and at subsequent visits, the tests will usually be done again to see if you have improved. You perform these simple and painless tests by breathing out as quickly and as completely as you can into a special machine, called a spirometer, after first filling your lungs with air as completely as possible. Such tests tell your doctor whether you have obstruction to airflow from the air passages. If the test is repeated after giving you a bronchodilator medi-

cation that opens up the airways, it is possible to tell to what extent the airway narrowing can be reversed by treatment. Such tests take only a few minutes in the doctor's surgery and can tell whether asthma is the most likely diagnosis, but only if, at the time of the visit, airway narrowing is actually present. Since some people with asthma have problems only at certain times of the year (such as in the pollen season) or under certain circumstances (such as with exercise), evidence that the condition is present may be lacking when you are actually seeing your doctor. Thus, your story of the illness is usually all-important! If airway narrowing is absent at that time but you and your doctor suspect asthma, special tests are available to confirm that you do have asthma (see *Chapter 9*).

If the asthma has been present for a long time and inflammatory changes in the airway, such as swelling, are severe, causing persistent airway narrowing, the response to bronchodilator medications may be poor when you are first tested. This may lead your doctor to suspect conditions such as chronic bronchitis or emphysema, which are usually much less correctable than asthma. It is for this reason that all patients with narrowed airways, thought to be suffering from chronic lung disease, are given 2 or 3 weeks of treatment with fairly large doses of anti-inflammatory steroid medications (prednisone or prednisolone) (also see *Chapter 11*) as part of the assessment. Asthma challenge tests (see *Chapter 9*) are helpful for establishing the presence and severity of the disease and need only be carried out if the simple breathing tests are almost normal at the time of testing.

MILD, MODERATE AND SEVERE ASTHMA

Understanding the severity of your asthma is extremely important because it enables you to anticipate when you will need to increase your treatment to avoid getting into really serious and perhaps life-threatening difficulty.

MILD ASTHMA

In mild asthma, inflammation of the airway lining is slight, breathlessness is usually mild, and wheezing attacks are infrequent and usually related mainly to certain triggers such as exercise or cold air exposure (see *Chapter 8*). There is, almost always, an excellent response to treatment with bronchodilator ("reliever") medication sprays that you administer to yourself before exertion or infrequently (not more than three or four times a week) when needed. These provide rapid and complete relief from breathlessness for several hours. In mild asthma, you have never had the need to go to a hospital emergency department or be admitted to hospital because of severe attacks.

Note: Even so-called mild asthma can become severe under certain circumstances, such as a viral infection of the air passages or exposure to a very large dose of allergen (e.g., running through a field of grass in midsummer or entering a house with many cats).

MODERATE ASTHMA

In moderate asthma, inflammation of the airway lining is more severe, symptoms that vary in severity from day to day are present most of the time, but are usually fairly mild to moderate and do not interfere with work or play, except perhaps in cold weather and on rare occasions when a chest cold may lead to increased difficulty. Awakening at night is unusual, visits to the hospital emergency department are very rare,

and hospitalization is rarely required, except perhaps when the asthma gets much worse due to the flu or a bad chest cold. With medication you can generally be kept free of symptoms most of the time, but in addition to the inhaled bronchodilator medications (used when needed), inhaled anti-inflammatory medications (see *Chapter 11*), such as cromoglycate and steroid sprays, are needed on a daily basis by adults and children. These medications **must** be taken daily even when your symptoms are not present in order to keep them from coming back. Treating asthma to **prevent** symptoms is like brushing your teeth every day to prevent tooth decay.

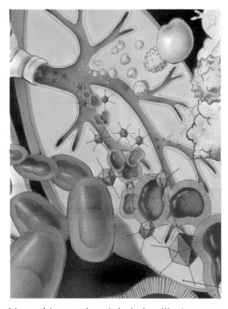

Many things, when inhaled, will trigger an asthma attack.

SEVERE ASTHMA

In severe asthma, the airways are very inflamed and irritable, symptoms are frequent and are made worse by trigger factors such as exercise and cold air and also by dusts, smoky rooms, car exhausts, paint fumes, household sprays, and perfume, etc. There is frequent awakening at night with wheezing or cough and often chest tightness, cough, and phlegm, when you get up in the morning. Asthma symptoms are extremely variable and frequently interfere with school, work, or sports activities. Visits to the hospital emergency department may be frequent, and repeat admissions to hospital, where you are given steroids intravenously or as tablets, may be necessary until the asthma is well controlled. If you have these features, you would be called a "brittle" asthmatic, and you are at high risk of serious life-threatening asthma episodes and at risk of dying of asthma. If you are in group 2 or 3, it is **essential** that you be put on so-called prophylactic (preventive) anti-inflammatory treatment in doses adequate to control the condition so as to return you to a relatively normal and complaint-free life (see *Chapter 11*).

CONTROL IS POSSIBLE

While it is not possible for **all** asthmatics to be symptom free all the time, the vast majority of people with asthma can lead normal lives free of asthma complaints with the excellent, presently available medicines, provided that these are **taken regularly, effectively**, and in **sufficient doses** to control the **inflammation** that is the basis of your asthma.

VARIATIONS ON THE THEME

Just as the saying "all that wheezes isn't asthma" contains more than a grain of truth, so it is that things that don't wheeze, such as persistent cough, may be asthma. The underlying cause is airway inflammation associated with airway irritability, usually with the production of excess secretions coughed up as phlegm. Your persistent cough may, like asthma, need treatment with inhaled anti-inflammatory agents and drugs nor-

mally used as bronchodilators to control it (see *Chapters 10 and 11*).

SO, DO I HAVE ASTHMA?

Answering the question "do I have asthma?" may be fairly straightforward if you complaints are absolutely characteristic. On the other hand, if the condition is less typical or if one of the look-alike conditions gives you complaints similar to those of asthma, it may be difficult for you and your doctor to make the diagnosis. Furthermore, conditions such as chronic bronchitis with airway narrowing, which commonly results from cigarette smoking for many years, or even regurgitation of stomach acid into your throat and aspiration of small amounts of this material into your lungs over long periods of time may confuse the issue and make the diagnosis of asthma very difficult indeed. You and your doctor working closely together should, through your careful description of complaints, together with analysis of the information, physical examination, and special tests requested by your doctor, achieve the correct diagnosis and treatment.

THE NOSE, THE EYES, AND ASTHMA

The nose can be thought of as the gatekeeper of the lungs. The nose filters, warms, and humidifies the incoming air and thus reduces possible irritation or injury to the lungs. Not surprisingly, the lining of the nose, which looks and acts much like the lining of the air passages in the lungs, is often affected in much the same way as the lungs in people with asthma. This condition, called *rhinitis*, is well known to many people who suffer from the grass pollen allergy called hay fever. Hay fever may cause itchiness of the throat and may be accompanied by asthma. Small pollen particles from trees or grass are

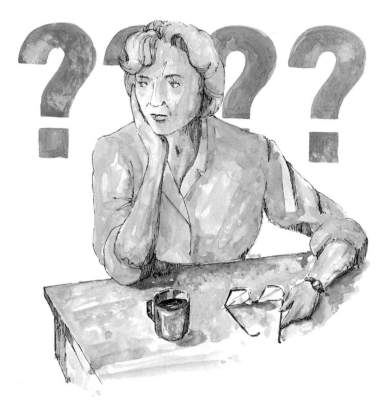

breathed into the lungs and often cause asthma.

The nose is also frequently involved in the nonallergic form of asthma. Nose problems, especially running, plugging, and spells of sinus infection (*sinusitis*) often occur for years before asthma develops. In the allergic form of asthma, there is almost always accompanying inflammation and irritation of the eyes, known as *conjunctivitis*. In fact, the presence of conjunctivitis is an important clue that the problem is allergic since the eyes are almost never involved in the nonallergic form of asthma, while the nose may be affected in both.

PERSISTENT COUGH: COULD IT BE ASTHMA?

Persistent cough is one of the most common symptoms of lung disease and often means that there is inflammation or irritation of the lining of the air passages. A persistent cough, sometimes with phlegm, may be one of the major features of asthma, particularly in children. Infants and children may have recurring episodes that last from a few days to a few weeks. These are often called "colds," particularly if the nose runs or plugs up as well. Such symptoms are most common at night, when they may awaken the child from sleep, and the cough may at times be so severe that children retch and vomit. In adults, cough may also be one of the most prominent features of the asthmatic condition and is sometimes associated with expectoration (or coughing up) of moderate amounts of clear or yellow phlegm (one or two tablespoonfuls a day) or occasionally fairly large amounts such as ½ to 1 oz. (30 to 50 ml).

Other possible causes of persistent cough include viral illnesses such as the whooping cough (*pertussis*). A cough may persist after a viral illness for several weeks or months if left untreated. If it does not improve steadily and disappear in 3 or 4 weeks, the possibility that the cough represents an asthma-like condition should be considered. It is important that a persistent cough be considered as possibly an asthma equivalent because the best treatment would then be like that for asthma (see *Chapter 11*).

No matter what the cause of the cough, cough suppressing medicines are not the best treatment and should never be used for more than a few days without consulting a doctor. No stone should be left unturned to try to establish the cause of persistent cough since, in addition to asthma, other causes may be present, including a postnasal (behind the nose) drip due to sinusitis; a foreign object, such as a peanut or chicken bone stuck in the airway after inadvertent inhalation; intermittent irritation of the lining of the airway by stomach juices that may be aspirated into the lungs, particularly at night; or more serious causes such as cancer of the lung, particularly in adults who have smoked about a packet a day for twenty or more years. The cause of the persistent cough can usually be determined with appropriate tests such as X-rays of the chest, sinuses, stomach, and oesophagus; challenge tests to see if the airways are excessively sensitive and "twitchy"; and allergy skin tests to determine whether the problem could relate to hypersensitivity (e.g., pets, house dust, pollens, moulds) (see *Chapter 9*).

Once the cause of the cough has been established, it is usually relatively simple to treat it effectively just like asthma and bring it under good control, or even cure it, depending on its cause.

If the cough persists in spite of an apparently well established diagnosis and potentially effective treatment, bronchoscopy should be used to look into the air passages in order to exclude such things as an inhaled foreign objects or an airway tumour.

7   All That Wheezes Isn't Asthma

AS YOU recall from *Chapter 6*, wheezing is a common symptom of asthma, although it may not be very prominent in some asthmatics. This is particularly true for small children, in whom ongoing or recurring episodes of cough (often called *bronchitis* or *bronchiolitis*) may be much more obvious or, indeed, the major symptom.

On the other hand, wheezing may appear in other conditions that may look like asthma at first and so may be treated as though asthma were present. There are four conditions that commonly mimic asthma:

1. Heart failure, most commonly a result of narrowing of the main arteries to the heart (ischaemic heart disease) or previous heart attack.
2. Inhaled objects may be the cause of the symptoms in children, but asthma-like symptoms sometimes occur in adults as well because of inhaling a peanut, a piece of plastic, a broken fragment of tooth, a chicken bone, etc. This may be a particular problem in the very elderly, who may have choking spells because of inhaling food during meals.
3. Food and acid regurgitation from the stomach into the gullet (oesophagus), sometimes with aspiration of small amounts of food or acid into the lung. This often happens when you are asleep.
4. Chronic bronchitis and emphysema mainly due to inhaling tobacco smoke for many years.

1. CONGESTIVE HEART FAILURE

This condition occurs most often in older people with known heart disease. People who suffer from heart failure have excessive fluid in their lungs, which narrows the airways by accumulating around them, and they may wheeze during such attacks. Typically attacks occur at night when lying flat, and so they must sit up to catch their breath. They often have accompanying chest tightness, and may also cough and raise a thin phlegm, sometimes with a pink tinge because it contains a small amount of blood. Asthma may be a possible diagnosis. Examination of the heart and lungs often reveals that the problem is primarily due to poor functioning of the heart.

Patients with this so-called "cardiac asthma" do not respond well to asthma medications but do respond well to those that strengthen heart function, reduce the load on the heart by opening up the arteries in the body, or decrease the overall amount of fluid in the body and in the lungs ("water pills").

2. INHALED OBJECTS

The fact that our swallowing and breathing functions partly share the same channel predisposes us to inhaling anything that gets into our mouth and throat. Thus young children may inhale anything they can get into their mouth. Nuts are a common culprit, and they should not be given to children under age 4. Nuts cause severe irritation and inflammation in the airway lining leading to cough, wheezing, infection (pneumonia), and sometimes complete obstruction of part of the airway, which may cause collapse of part of the lung. In adults, pieces of tooth may come loose and be inhaled under anaesthetic during theatre work. Foodstuffs such as small poultry bones may be inhaled, particularly if coughing is impaired by alcohol or by "nerve" pills or sleeping pills. The resulting airway blockage and increased secretions may cause symptoms similar to asthma. Again, failure to respond to asthma treatment is the clue that asthma is not present; this should lead to additional investigations, including inspection of your air passages by bronchoscopy.

3. REFLUX OF STOMACH CONTENTS AND STOMACH JUICE ASPIRATION

In the disorder doctors call gastro-oesophageal reflux, stomach contents may pass up into the gullet (oesophagus), particularly when you are sleeping. This may cause irritation of the oesophagus and sometimes lead to inhalation of small amounts of food and stomach acid. Because the cough reflex is blunted when you are asleep, the inhaled acid and food particles may not cause much cough at the time. Damage to the air passages and lungs and failure to clear out the foreign material may lead to pneumonia, which may recur. This may result in badly damaged lungs due to scarring (*fibrosis*) or destruction of the airway lining and wall (*bronchiectasis*). If the cough reflex is fairly active, you may be awakened by violent coughing or choking. The choking may result from the vocal cords going into spasm when they are irritated, similar to the experience of laughing while eating or drinking. Inhaling small amounts of stomach contents only once or twice a week will cause typical chronic bron-

chitis. With time, the resulting inflammation of the airway leads to airway narrowing and causes most of the symptoms of asthma.

Once again, the clue that this is not asthma comes from the failure to respond to asthma treatment, and this will often lead your doctor to inquire more about heartburn and indigestion. Other clues are coughing and acid or food regurgitation or choking spells. Occasionally spasm of the vocal cords leading to noisy breathing called "stridor" occurs on inhalation when you are awakened from sleep.

This condition is usually treated by reducing the likelihood that acid and food particles will get into your lungs. This can be done by elevating the head of the bed 10 to 14 cm (4 to 6 inches) on blocks, since piling up pillows is rarely effective, and avoiding alcohol, coffee, tea, and chocolate, particularly in the evening. People with this problem are advised to avoid eating within 4 to 5 hours before going to bed and achieve their ideal weight if they are overweight. They are also given medications to speed the emptying of food from the stomach and reduce the production and acidity of digestive juices.

4. CHRONIC BRONCHITIS AND EMPHYSEMA

These are inflammatory conditions of the airways and lungs that commonly coexist. They are usually a result of heavy smoking (10 to 20 cigarettes a day for 20 or 30 years). The cigarette smoke damages the airway walls and causes an overproduction of secretions. Eventually the airways become narrowed permanently in about 25 percent of smokers. If you have asthma and also inhale tobacco smoke, you will add a second insult to the underlying injury caused by the asthma. This often leads to very severe and irreversible airway narrowing and damage to your air passages.

Is Your Wheezing Cough or Breathlessness due to Asthma?

Checklist	There can be considerable variability in the symptoms.	Yes	No

- Coughing and wheezing at night that you can't shake off or that keeps coming back
- Tightness in the chest, wheezing, or breathlessness in cold weather particularly during exercise
- "Chestiness" that does not get better after 4 weeks following an attack of flu
- "Wheezy bronchitis" after a cold
- Your child wakes often at night coughing
- Greater than usual breathlessness after running for a bus or playing sports
- Tightness in the chest and breathlessness that develops after ingesting certain foods
- Breathlessness after taking aspirin, certain arthritis medicines, certain heart medicines, or glaucoma eye drops

If **any** of the above are "**yes**," ask your doctor; you might have asthma!

TABLE 7–1 COMPARISON OF SYMPTOMS OF ASTHMA, CHRONIC BRONCHITIS, EMPHYSEMA, AND HEART FAILURE

Symptoms	Asthma	Chronic Bronchitis	Emphysema	Heart Failure
• Cough	+++	+++	+−o	++−o
• Phlegm production	++	+++	+−o	+−o
• Phlegm colour	yellow*/ clear	clear/ yellow**	clear/ yellow**	clear or pink***
• Variability of breathlessness and wheeze	++++	+	o−+	o−++
• Daytime breathlessness	o−++++	o−++++	o−++++	o−+++
• Nightime breathlessness	o−++++	o−++	o	+−++++
• Exercise breathlessness	+++−++++	+−++++	++++	++++
• Nasal obstruction (rhinitis)	o−++++	o	o	o
• Eye irritation (conjunctivitis)	o−++++	o	o	o

o = not present   +−++++ = mild to severe
* In asthma, the yellow colour may be caused by eosinophils or infection.
** In chronic bronchitis and emphysema, the yellow colour always means that the phlegm is infected.
*** The pink colour is due to blood.
Diagnosis of asthma may be difficult since other conditions may mimic it.

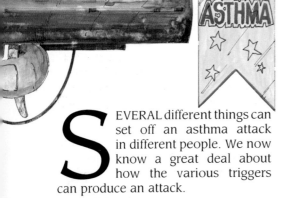

8   Asthma Triggers

SEVERAL different things can set off an asthma attack in different people. We now know a great deal about how the various triggers can produce an attack.

ALLERGIC FACTORS

An asthma attack can be triggered by breathing in an allergic substance or *allergen*, such as grass pollen grains, house dust, or certain mould spores. Wheezing may begin within a few minutes of exposure and is caused by triggering of mast cells, as discussed in *Chapter 5*. People given an allergen mist to inhale in the laboratory commonly have an immediate attack of wheezing that recovers within 1 to 2 hours, but it may be followed by a later attack about 6 hours after the exposure. Furthermore, the next day the airways are more twitchy, and this increased sensitivity of the air passages may go on for about 2 weeks. It is now known that the late onset wheeze and the increased twitchiness are caused by increased inflammation of the lining of the airways with eosinophils and damage to the lining, as discussed in *Chapter 5*. This means that continued exposure to the allergic factor produces a grumbling, long-lasting inflammation of the airways.

This is what happens during the pollen season, when the airways become more inflamed and twitchy, leading to more frequent symptoms. This explains why avoiding allergic factors is so important. Of course, it is difficult completely to avoid exposure to certain things, such as house dust. In an experiment in which volunteers were kept in a dust-free environment for 2 months, their asthma became much better, and the twitchiness of their airways went away. Such extreme measures are not practical at home, but even simple measures to reduce house dust mites in the bedroom may help (see p. 147). If such measures are less than completely effective, drug treatment may be needed, as discussed in *Chapters 10 and 11*.

The most common allergens are:

1. **House dust mite**, which occurs throughout the year.
2. **Pollen**, which occurs at various times depending on the season: tree pollens in spring, weed and grass pollens in summer, and, in North America, ragweed in autumn. Flower pollens do not normally give any problems.

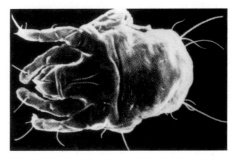

A house dust mite as seen by the electron microscope.

3. **Mould spores**, which usually occur in the autumn, but can be found at any time of the year.
4. **Family pets**, including cats, dogs, horses, rabbits, hamsters, gerbils, mice and rats, can also cause an allergic reaction. Exposure to these allergic factors can also lead to a runny nose and itchy eyes, as discussed in *Chapter 15*.

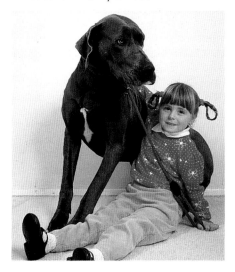

EXERCISE

Wheezing, with chest tightness and undue breathlessness, that comes on after exercise or exertion, is very common. It is particularly noticeable in children, but only because they run more than adults. Sudden bursts of running are the worst for triggering wheezing. Usually the wheezing begins, or gets worse for a few minutes, after stopping running, although it may start during the run. This is called exercise-induced asthma which can be shown in the laboratory by getting a patient to run on a treadmill or ride an exercise bike. The level of exercise is set to bring on wheezing, which can be shown by a fall in measured peak expired flow (PEF) values (see peak flow test, *Chapter 9*) after exercise. This is sometimes used as a test of asthma

in children, in whom exercise may be the only trigger. Strangely enough, continuing the exercise may cause the asthma to gradually improve, and many asthmatics have noticed that they can "run through" their asthma. The reason for this is that exercise causes the blood level of adrenaline, a natural hormone produced by the adrenal glands, to go up, and this is a good bronchodilator (reliever of asthma).

Why do asthmatics get wheezy when they exercise while non-asthmatics don't? This question has puzzled researchers for many years, but recently the answers are becoming clearer. When people exercise, breathing becomes faster and deeper. This leads to drying out of the delicate lining of the airways. If people with exercise-induced asthma sit down and over-breathe exactly the same amount as during exercise, they develop a similar degree of wheezing because the drying out of the airways is the same. If they breathe dry air (rather than normal air that contains a certain amount of water vapour), then the wheezing is more severe and occurs sooner because the airways dry out even more quickly. On the other hand, if they breathe in air that is very humid, the wheezing is less severe. These experiments fit in with what some asthmatic patients have discovered, namely that running in cold, dry weather is more likely to bring on wheezing than in warm, humid weather. Also, breathing through the nose, rather than through the mouth, causes less wheezing because the air breathed in is then humidified more. Swimming is less likely to cause asthma than running, possibly because the air close to the water surface is more humid, and so this reduces the drying out effect.

Paradoxically, however, some asthmatics find that their asthma symptoms are more troublesome in humid weather. The reason why is not well understood, but is probably the result of allergens, which favour humid conditions (eg moulds), rather than the humidity itself.

There are two theories as to how drying out of the airways produces wheezing and both are probably correct. First, when the airways dry out they cool as water evaporates and, second, drying out of the airways means that the thin layer of liquid that coats the airway lining becomes more concentrated. Both of these may trigger the mast cells at the airway surface to release chemicals that cause bronchospasm. Exercise-induced asthma may be prevented by using a bronchodilator before exercise (this prevents the muscle from going into spasm) or preventative medication that reduces the likelihood that the mast cells will release their chemicals (see *Chapter 5*).

LAUGHTER

Some asthmatics notice that they get wheezy when they laugh. The cause is similar to the exercise-induced asthma already discussed. Laughing is associated with sudden rapid intake of breath, which may cause drying out of the airways. It is particularly seen in asthmatics with a high degree of twitchiness. It is an annoying symptom, but it can be blocked by

treatments similar to those for exercise-induced asthma.

WEATHER

Many asthmatics notice that certain types of weather make their asthma worse, and particularly changes in the weather. There may be several reasons for this. A sudden change in temperature can trigger wheezing. Going from a warm house into the cold commonly brings on wheezing, presumably because of cooling of the airways (as discussed above). Conversely, going from outside into a hot room, or the onset of hot weather, may also lead to increased wheezing. Asthma does not seem to be any more common in cold climates than in hot weather, however, and the weather does not seem to greatly affect the amount of asthma in a community. However, there are variations between individuals and some asthmatics find they are worse at a particular time of year. This may be due to associated events (eg colds) rather than to temperature.

The weather can also affect asthma by increasing the allergens in the atmosphere. In the pollen season, people allergic to grass pollen are worse after a dry spell because the pollen count is higher. Sometimes unusual weather can trigger asthma. Asthma attacks have been related to

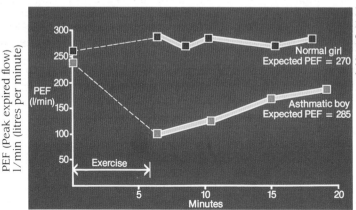

Peak flow chart following exercise comparing the PEF of a normal girl and an asthmatic boy.

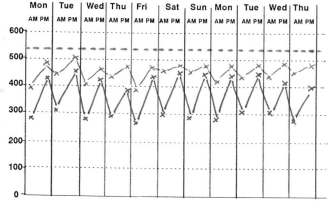

| Mon | Tue | Wed | Thu | Fri | Sat | Sun | Mon | Tue | Wed | Thu |

Peak flow chart of a patient with asthma showing marked variation in peak flow over the day, with low values in the early morning and higher values in the evening. This patient noticed tightness of the chest on waking every morning and awoke very early 3–4 times per week because of asthma symptoms. Blue lines show peak flow values before taking an inhaler, and red lines show values after taking two puffs of salbutamol inhaler. Green dotted lines show the expected values for someone of the same age, sex and height without asthma.

heavy rain after a thunderstorm, which resulted in the release of mould spores to which people were allergic. In Australia, storms have been shown to rupture pollen grains, which may increase symptoms in pollen-sensitive asthmatics.

WHEEZING AT NIGHT

Worsening of asthma at night is extremely common. In a recent survey, as many as 80 percent of patients had an episode of wheezing at night at least once a week. Asthmatics characteristically wake between 3:00 to 5:00 A.M., and may do so for several nights in a row, especially when the asthma is bad. Many asthmatics get so used to waking at night that they think it is normal, and don't even bother to tell the doctor. However, it is troublesome, since disturbed sleep may interfere with daytime activities, particularly in children. Wheezing at night is *always* a sign of asthma that is out of control and indicates the need for more preventive (rather than bronchodilator) treatment. Although asthma may be well controlled in the daytime, wheezing in the early hours of the morning may lead to wakening.

The reason asthmatics wheeze at night is still not certain, but there are many theories. In the sixteenth century, Sir Thomas Willis wrote that overheating of the blood by the bedclothes was the likely cause. Exposure to allergic factors in bedding (such as feathers or house dust) may be responsible in some people, but cannot explain why wheezing gets worse in asthmatics who are not allergic. Other theories include the possibility that lying down may make the airways narrower (but the increased wheeze comes on several hours after going to sleep) or that acid from the stomach gets into the gullet and somehow stimulates increased wheezing. Sleep itself may be a contributing factor, but in a study where asthmatics were kept awake at night, increased wheezing still came on in the early hours.

Perhaps the most plausible explanation is that several bodily functions show a 24-hour variation, called a *circadian rhythm*. Circadian means literally "about a day," indicating that the fluctuation occurs over a 24-hour period. These rhythms are coordinated by a special "timer" in the brain. The size of the airways also shows a variation and, in normal people, the airways get narrower in the early hours of the morning, although the degree of narrowing is so slight that it is not noticeable. However, in asthmatics the degree of narrowing is much greater, and is related to the degree of airway twitchiness. The increased airway narrowing may be related to a decrease in the levels of adrenaline and cortisone in the bloodstream and an increase in activity of bronchoconstrictor nerves. There is also evidence that the amount of inflammation increases at night. All these factors combine to produce a marked increase in the wheeze in asthmatics. It follows that treatment of wheezing at night involves not only long-acting bronchodilator preparations to prevent the airway narrowing, but, even more important, overall reduction of the inflammation, which appears to be a critical factor leading to exaggeration of the normally unnoticed rhythm.

INFECTIONS

Asthmatics often get worse during a chest infection, and infections are frequently the cause of bad attacks of asthma. These infections are often caused by a **virus**, and the reason certain virus infections (like flu) are particularly troublesome in asthmatics is that they damage the lining of the airways. As we learned earlier, this is already a site of trouble in asthma. The effects of a virus infection may last for weeks, as it may take this long for the lining of the airway to heal. Again, inflammation triggered by the virus that is the problem, and anti-inflammatory drugs work best to clear it up (see *Chapters 10 and 11*). Infections with bacteria are very uncommon triggers of asthma, so antibiotics that kill bacteria are rarely of much benefit in asthma attacks, unless infection caused by bacteria is also present. Sinus infections may also contribute to asthma deterioration and should be treated.

STRESS

Stress and anxiety do not "cause" asthma, but these are common triggering factors in some patients. This is discussed in more detail in *Chapter 19*.

ASPIRIN AND AETHRITIS MEDICINES

In a small proportion of asthmatics, taking aspirin can trigger a severe attack within 15 to 20 minutes. Less than one percent of asthmatics are aspirin-sensitive, and they are almost always older asthmatics who do not have an obvious allergic predisposition. Sinus problems and polyps in the nose are often seen in this group of asthmatics. Even a single tablet of aspirin can cause a severe attack, which often starts with flushing of the face and a running nose, followed by wheezing.

The reason aspirin affects this small group of asthmatics is not yet fully understood, but other drugs that work in the same way as aspirin (known as nonsteroidal anti-inflammatory drugs or NSAIDs), by blocking the production of certain natural chemicals called prostaglandins, have a similar effect. All of this group of drugs, which are usually used as pain killers in arthritis or to prevent blood clotting, need to be **carefully avoided** in susceptible asthmatics. It is important to be aware of which drugs to avoid, and to realize that many treatments for colds that do not require a doctor's prescription may contain aspirin. So, it is always important to check carefully whether any treatment you take contains aspirin. If taking these medicines causes asthma attacks and you develop joint problems (arthritis), so that these medicines are essential to control pain and stiffness, your doctor can arrange for you to see a specialist who can desensitize you by starting with **very** small doses of aspirin and then slowly increasing the dose to adequate levels.

9   Testing for Asthma

SEVERAL tests may be performed to evaluate asthma, and these are done for a variety of reasons:

1. To diagnose asthma
2. To give an indication of severity of asthma
3. To assess the response to treatment
4. Occasionally for research into new treatments, etc.

ALLERGY SKIN TEST

Because asthma is most often caused by allergies, you may be given an allergy skin test. This is a simple test in which a drop of allergen solution is placed on the skin of the forearm and the skin is slightly and painlessly pricked with a needle. If you are allergic, the skin becomes itchy after 5 minutes, a small blister forms, and the surrounding area becomes reddened. Usually a number of allergic extracts (12 to 20) are tested at the same time, including pollens, house dust mite, cat and dog, moulds, and sometimes certain foods. It is then possible to see which factors you are allergic to. The skin reactions go down within an hour.

Often several skin tests come up positive, but some reactions are bigger than others. This does not necessarily mean that they are more important in asthma. Indeed, even people without allergic conditions may have positive skin tests. The factors that you have noticed to be associated with asthma symptoms (for example, contact with cats) are the most important in establishing that your asthma is caused by allergies. Some people with asthma, usually those whose asthma develops after the age of 40, have no skin re-

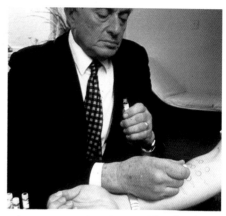

Skin tests can pinpoint specific allergies.

actions since they do not have an obvious allergy. The cause of this non-allergic form of asthma is still a mystery although, from the way it begins, virus infection seems likely.

CHEST X-RAY

In asthma, the chest X-ray is usually routine and is done to make sure there are no other conditions present as well. Occasionally, asthmatics have shadows on the X-ray: these are usually because of plugs of phlegm blocking the air passages, which may be caused by an allergic reaction to certain mould spores. The X-ray of asthmatics, particularly when they have a severe attack, may show the lungs to be excessively blown up with trapped air.

BREATHING TESTS

Several tests measure how much the air passages are narrowed: these tests measure the amount of air that can be forcibly blown out of the lungs. In

49

asthma, as the air passages become obstructed it takes longer to breathe the air out of your lungs (like trying to force air through a straw). It is possible to measure this using a machine called a *spirometer*. You breathe in as deeply as you can and then blow out as quickly as possible — the amount of air breathed out in 1 second (a test called, not surprisingly, the "one second forced expired volume" or FEV_1 for short) then gives a measurement of how relatively narrow the airways are, because the value obtained is compared with normal values from people of the same age, sex, and height. (As you might expect, the larger the size of the ribcage and chest, the larger the volume of air that can be breathed out.) The total amount of air breathed out until the lungs are empty can also be measured — this may also be reduced in asthma. One of the best tests of asthma is to see whether these results improve after a bronchodilator (reliever) is used. This demonstrates the *reversibility* or improvement of the airway narrowing, which is one of the important features of asthma.

Sometimes more complicated lung function tests are done. These might incude tests in which you sit in a box like a telephone booth and breathe through a mouthpiece. In this way your doctor can measure more detailed aspects of lung function. This can be helpful in trying to distinguish asthma from other lung conditions.

PEAK FLOW METERS AND CHARTS

One of the most useful tests of all in asthma is the peak flow test, because it is simple and cheap. The measuring device, which reliably measures airway narrowing, is easily carried around. It can be used at home or at work, and the measurement takes only a minute. Measuring lung function only once in the surgery, with even the most sophisticated equipment, may

not show what the asthma is really like because airway narrowing varies so much from time to time. Many asthmatics are worst during the night or first thing in the morning and improve during the day (even without treatment). So if you are seen in a clinic in the afternoon, tests of lung function may be normal, suggesting to your doctor that asthma is not present or is much milder than it really is.

A peak flow meter measures the speed with which air can be blown out of the lungs. You fill your lungs as much as possible and then, after putting your lips around the mouthpiece, you blow all the air out as fast as you can. You then simply read the value on the scale. As a rule, it is best to blow three times and to only use the highest value (to allow for bad blows). Usually you will be asked to measure peak flow first thing in the morning and last thing at night, before and after using your bronchodilator (reliever) inhaler. The values obtained can either be written on a piece of paper or, preferably, marked down on a chart. It is then possible to see how severe the asthma becomes and how it changes with time. When the asthma is more severe, many patients find that the early morning value is lower than the evening value — this "morning dip" reflects increased airway narrowing at night.

Using peak flow charts, it is possible to see how you respond to various treatments. A particularly useful test in some patients is to see if and how much the peak flow improves with a 2- or 3-week course of steroid tablets. This is because some asthmatics, especially if their asthma has been poorly controlled for a long time, improve only after many days of steroid tablets and do not show much immediate improvement in peak flow after using a bronchodilator inhaler. Peak flow charts are also useful in testing new

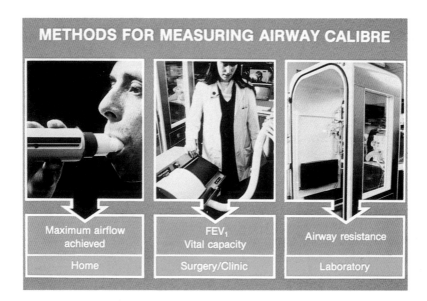

METHODS FOR MEASURING AIRWAY CALIBRE

Maximum airflow achieved	FEV₁ Vital capacity	Airway resistance
Home	Surgery/Clinic	Laboratory

asthma treatments, and your doctor may ask you to help with a research study. By assisting with such research, you may help in the development of new and better treatments for yourself and other asthmatics.

EXERCISE TESTS

Occasionally an exercise test is helpful, particularly in children. As discussed in *Chapter 8*, exercise commonly triggers an attack of wheezing. This can be simulated in the laboratory by running on a treadmill or performing bicycle exercise. The degree of exercise can then be carefully controlled and measurements of lung function (with a spirometer or peak flow meter) done. This test may be useful in children who only have symptoms of asthma on exercise and whose lung function tests are otherwise normal.

ASTHMA PROVOCATION OR CHALLENGE TESTS

Asthma challenge tests are often useful, usually when there is a strong suspicion of asthma but the other tests are normal. These tests measure the degree of twitchiness of the airways (which relates to how inflamed the airways are at the time of testing).

The test is done by inhaling a mist of a substance that causes mild bronchospasm. Usually either histamine (a natural chemical mediator already discussed) or methacholine (a chemical that also constricts airway muscle) are used. After measuring lung function (by spirometer or peak flow meter), you breathe in a mist (usually from a nebulizer, or atomizer) for a couple of minutes, and then lung function tests are repeated. The amount of active substance in the mist is then gradually increased and the test repeated again. This goes on until your air passages narrow a little, lung function begins to fall, and you begin to feel a little wheezy or tight. This test then gives a measurement of the amount of the challenge substance needed to cause a certain degree of bronchospasm – in other words, it measures the increased sensitivity or twitchiness in the airways. The greater the twitchiness, the smaller the amount of provoking substance needed. The more twitchy the airways are, the more severe is the asthma and the more anti-inflammatory (preventer) medication will be needed to control the disease.

Sometimes patients with asthma are given an aerosol of an allergic factor (e.g., pollen extracts or industrial chemicals) to which they may be allergic, and the same test is done. This is not a routine test but is very useful for finding the cause of asthma, especially in job-related asthma (see *Chapter 16*). It is also useful in research into new treatments, as the beneficial effect of drugs on asthma can be studied.

HOME MONITORING

Just as measuring blood pressure is the best way to be sure that treatment is working well for high blood pressure (hypertension) and measuring blood sugar is used by diabetics to be sure that diabetes is under good control, so measuring the peak flow is the best way to be sure that your asthma is under the best possible control. This test acts as an early warning of deterioration and allows you to make adjustments in your medication, before the situation becomes serious.

1. The peak flow helps to establish the **pattern** of asthma, which assists you and your doctor in selecting the right treatment and adjusting the dose to keep you as well controlled as possible.
2. The peak flow may reveal that your asthma is in fact more or less severe than you or your doctor think. Many of the symptoms of asthma are not specific and could come from other coexisting conditions. For example, Jennifer, diagnosed as a severe asthmatic was having a lot of chest tightness, which she interpreted as deterioration of the disease. This resulted in repeated short courses of prednisolone pills, without much relief. When she visited her doctor, he did spirometry and found the tests to be normal. This made him think that perhaps the symptom of chest tightness was unrelated to asthma, and he therefore asked her to record the peak flow regularly,

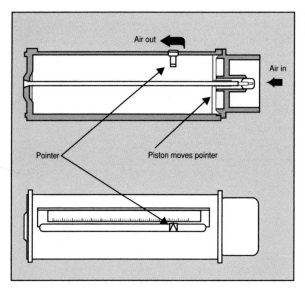

Cross-sectional view of a peak flow meter.

Air out

Air in

Pointer

Piston moves pointer

52

and particularly when the chest tightness was present. When she visited her doctor about 2 weeks later, she was able to show that, at times when the chest was tight, the peak flow was normal, ruling out asthma as a cause. It turned out that she had pain coming from her oesophagus (gullet), resulting from acid regurgitating from the stomach, which can cause a feeling of tightness similar to that experienced by asthmatics, rather than the usual heartburn. With the correct treatment for the reflux problem, she lost the chest tightness and is now feeling well.

3. Peak flow charts provide a record for the patient and the doctor over a period of time, which assures that control of the asthma is adequate. It also tells the patient early in the course of deterioration that control is not as good as it was and that additional medication is required. For example, Michele was feeling well, but the peak flow that she had been measuring regularly for many months, and which had remained in the range of 450 to 500 litres per minute (L/min), was gradually decreasing to 400, then 350 L/min, with few additional symptoms. At the same time, the variability in the peak flow increased, so that sometimes the peak flow was around 350, but at other times it was around 500. The reduction in the absolute peak flow value and the increase in the variability in the peak flow from time to time indicates poor control. Because she had been instructed to double the inhaled steroids when the value got to 350 or below, she did so, and within 3 to 4 days the peak flow was again back to 450.

4. Peak flows provide numbers that allow your doctor to give you precise instructions as to what you should do as the peak flow deteriorates (reflecting an increase in the airflow obstruction owing to increased swelling of the walls of your airways and/or spasm of the smooth muscle). Thus, if your usual peak flow is 500, and it remains 20

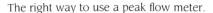

The right way to use a peak flow meter.

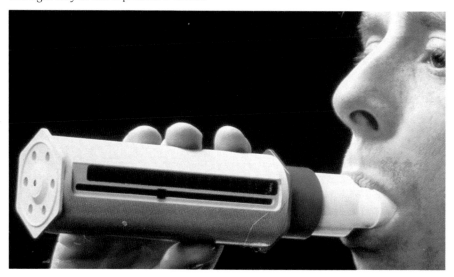

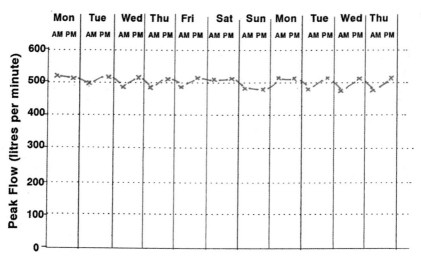

Peak flow of a person without asthma showing normal values throughout the day with little variation over the week.

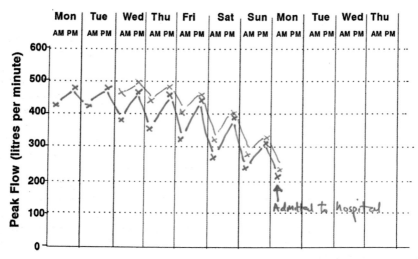

Peak flow chart of an asthmatic showing deterioration following the development of a cold. Peak flow falls progressively over a week. Response to the rescue bronchodilator also became less. The patient was admitted to hospital for treatment.

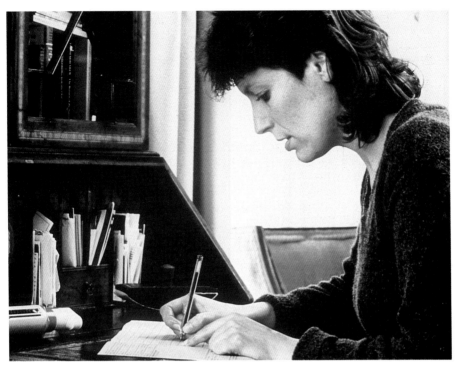
Monitor and record your peak flow readings on a daily basis.

percent below that at 400 L/min for 2 days in a row and does not increase to at least 450 after your usual bronchodilator medication (such as Ventolin, Berotec, or Bricanyl), your doctor would probably instruct you to double the dose of inhaled steroid. For example, if you were taking 2 puffs of Becotide four times a day to control the asthma, you would increase the dose to 4 puffs of Becotide four times a day for 1 to 2 weeks, and then resume the lower dose 1 week after your peak flow had returned to its "usual" level. If the peak flow drops by 30 percent to 350 L/min, you would begin taking prednisolone tablets (see *Chapters 11 and 12*) and continue these as instructed until the peak flow is again over 450, after which time the prednisolone would be rapidly tapered to zero or the previous maintenance level. If the peak flow falls by 40 percent or more to 300 or below, you would contact your doctor or go to the nearest hospital emergency room for treatment. On the way to the hospital, you would take 100 mg of prednisolone and bronchodilator puffs, as described in detail in *Chapter 12*. You would then follow your doctor's instructions as to how long to take the prednisolone and when to begin reducing it, as well as what level to maintain (if any) once you are well.

5. Peak flow measurements allow you to monitor that you are, in fact, maintaining good control of your asthma and normal function while treatment levels are gradually decreased, so that your doctor can determine the **minimum medication needed**.

6. It is not necessary for you to measure peak flow all the time once you are confident that the asthma is under control and your symptoms accurately inform you about the severity of the airway narrowing. Thus, you may wish to measure the peak flow for 2 or 3 months when the asthma diagnosis has first been established and after that only check it once or twice a week, except when you are more breathless. At those times, you should go back to measuring it regularly twice a day or more before and after your bronchodilator medication. Furthermore, if you have attacks from time to time, it is a good idea to record the peak flow to see how severe they are, how much variation there is from your usual values, and how much response you get to treatment.

If the values for peak flow are low (more than 15 percent below the usual values after you have taken your bronchodilator puffs), if the variation from measurement to measurement is greater (more than about 20 percent difference between the morning and night values), or if you get a poor response to the bronchodilator, your asthma is out of control and requires additional treatment (see *Chapter 12*).

In summary, if you combine the measurement of the peak flow with your symptoms, you should be able to establish whether you are under good control or not and make the necessary adjustments in your treatment.

If you follow the action plan described in *Chapter 11* but do not seem to be improving rapidly, you should contact your doctor or go to the nearest hospital casualty department for help.

10 How Asthma Treatments Work

A BEWILDERING number of treatments are now available for asthma, but the most effective way of treating the condition is more simple than it may first seem. This chapter describes some of the common treatments and how they work. *Chapters 11 and 12* discuss how you should use these treatments in controlling your asthma.

AN OUNCE OF PREVENTION...

Avoiding factors that will injure and inflame airways and triggers that are known to set off asthma is obviously helpful. This is particularly true for established allergic factors: avoiding exposure to pollen by not going out into fields during times of high pollen counts, reducing the amount of house dust, particularly in the bedroom, avoiding feather pillows and using artificial fillings for pillows and mattresses, damp dusting, regular vacuum cleaning, and replacing carpets by linoleum or other smooth surfaces on the floor may all be useful. However, it is not possible to eliminate the house dust mite completely by these measures. Chemical sprays that kill the house dust mite are not yet very successful while paint, which is claimed to kill these mites, is of no use. Eliminating the house dust mite is possible only with great difficulty, but where this has been done under special hospital conditions, there is a marked improvement in house dust sensitive patients with asthma. Interestingly, the house dust mite does not live at

'CURABLE' ASTHMA

MEDICINES
e.g. β–blockers, analgesics

SINGLE AVOIDABLE ALLERGEN
e.g. pets

OCCUPATION
e.g. welder, printer

Some avoidable factors which can trigger asthma.

high altitudes and where it is not humid, which explains why some asthmatics get better in the high mountains, such as the Swiss Alps or the Rockies. Avoiding chemicals at work that cause asthma is very important and special precautions must be taken (see *Chapter 16*).

Avoiding certain asthma triggers, such as exercise, would obviously reduce the symptoms but, if asthma is treated properly, it is almost always possible for the asthmatic to run (and laugh) normally. Asthma should not prevent normal activities, and the proper amount of treatment should be given to control the disease so that this is possible. Indeed, several Olympic athletes are asthmatic, showing what is possible. See page 146 to 149 for a detailed list of control measures.

INFLUENZA VACCINATION

Each winter season influenza virus infections lead to more or less serious epidemics of bronchitis and pneumonia. If you have asthma, such infections are likely to cause it to flare up and make you much sicker than non-asthmatic friends and colleagues, even to the point of a life-threatening attack. You should try to stay clear of people with the, flu although this may be virtually impossible. To protect yourself as much as possible you should see your family doctor **every autumn** for influenza vaccine, particularly if your asthma is severe.

ASTHMA TREATMENTS

INHALERS VS TABLETS OR LIQUIDS

Asthma treatments can be given by an inhaler directly into the lungs or in tablet form by mouth. In fact, usually the same treatment can be given either way, so why use one rather than the other?

ADVANTAGES OF INHALERS

Inhaled drugs are breathed directly into the airways so they usually act quickly (at least for bronchodilators), which is important if you need rapid relief of symptoms. It is also possible to use small doses to achieve a good effect – doses that are so small they do not get absorbed sufficiently into the body to cause unwanted effects. Inhalers are also easy to carry around and use when needed. Another advantage that has recently been recognized is that inhalers have a much better anti-asthma effect than the tablet form of the same treatment – possibly because the inhaled drug is able to reach certain cells lining the airway that are important in triggering attacks, as discussed in *Chapter 5*. This is particularly so in protecting against wheezing produced by trigger factors like exercise and allergens. Inhaler treatments are generally cheaper than tablets in the long run.

DISADVANTAGES OF INHALERS

The disadvantage of inhalers is that some people (especially small children and the elderly) find them difficult to use. However, new types of inhaler and add-on devices have been developed that make inhalers easy to use and provide other benefits as well (see *Chapter 13*). Another disadvantage is that inhaled bronchodilators may not last as long as the slow-release tablet forms and so may not be as effective in stopping the wheezing that comes on overnight. However, inhalers containing much longer-acting bronchodilators, lasting 12 hours or more, are now available in some countries. Furthermore, with well-controlled asthma (see *Chapter 11*) night-time symptoms should not be a problem.

ADVANTAGES AND DISADVANTAGES OF TABLETS

Tablet forms of many asthma treatments often have the great disadvantage of unwanted effects because, when taken by mouth in doses that relieve asthma, they have effects on other parts of the body. This limits the dose that can be given. Some asthma treatments, like theophylline, can **only** be given in tablet form and, because of the side effects, it is a poor first-choice treatment for asthma. Another disadvantage of tablets is the slow onset of effect. The advantage of tablet treatments is that long-acting forms are available that slowly release the drug from the stomach, so they may assist in treating night-time symptoms. Also, they are easy to take.

INHALED VERSUS ORAL
A SUMMARY

	INHALED	ORAL
DOSE	LOW	HIGH
SPEED OF ONSET	RAPID	SLOW
SIDE EFFECTS	FEW	MANY
ADMINISTRATION	REQUIRES INSTRUCTION	EASY
LENGTH OF ACTION	5-6h	5-6h
SITE OF ACTION	DIRECT	INDIRECT
PREVENTION OF EXERCISE ASTHMA	GOOD	POOR

INHALED VERSUS ORAL
SIDE EFFECTS OF BRONCHODILATORS

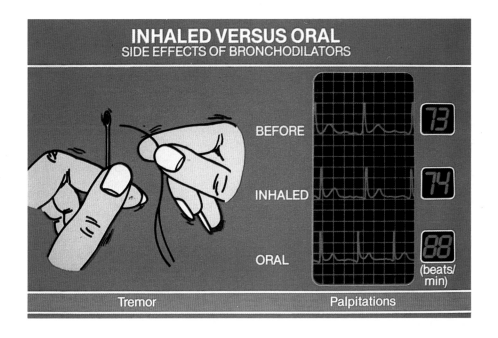

BEFORE 73

INHALED 74

ORAL 88 (beats/min)

Tremor   Palpitations

ASTHMA TREATMENT: RELIEVERS AND PREVENTERS

The treatments for asthma can be divided into two main groups: bronchodilators that relieve wheeze (the **relievers**), and anti-inflammatory drugs that work to reduce the inflammation of the airways (the **preventers**). The preventers should be used in a quite different way from bronchodilators and it is therefore important to understand what the different medicines do.

BRONCHODILATORS – THE ASTHMA RELIEVERS

There are only three types of bronchodilator drug:
1. Sympathomimetics (adrenaline-like substances)
2. Theophylline (a caffeine-like substance)
3. Anticholinergics (atropine-like substances)

However, there are many brand names, so it is often confusing.

1. SYMPATHOMIMETICS

These bronchodilators are all derived initially from adrenaline, the hormone released from a gland above the kidneys (adrenal gland) during stress. Drugs that act like adrenaline are called symphathomimetics because they mimic this hormone which is a part of the *sympathetic* (or "fight and flight") nervous system that responds to stress.

ADRENALINE

Adrenaline itself was first used as an asthma treatment at the beginning of this century. It was tried on asthma because it was known to blanch the skin, and it was believed that asthma was caused by congestion or engorgement of the lining of the air passages. (This theory has become popular again!) Adrenaline proved to be remarkably effective and gave rapid relief of symptoms when given by injection. But it could not be given by mouth, only lasted about an hour, and caused side effects such as heart palpitations. It is still used in many countries as a treatment for severe attacks, particularly in infants and children.

IMPROVING ADRENALINE: BETA AGONISTS

In the 1940s, German chemists improved upon adrenaline by chemically altering its structure to produce isoprenaline, which had fewer side effects. It was very effective as a bronchodilator when given by an inhaler and gave rapid relief. Isoprenaline is classified by doctors as a beta-agonist, because it works by stimulating "beta-receptors" on the special muscles in the walls of the air passages which cause these muscles to relax when activated (agonist means stimulator). This opens the narrowed air passages. Beta-receptors are named after the Greek letter beta, to distinguish them from alpha-receptors, which usually have the opposite effect. But beta-receptors are also found in the heart, so the disadvantage of isoprenaline was that it also caused palpitations and a racing heart. Also, like adrenaline, its benefits did not last more than about 30 minutes.

BETA 2 SELECTIVE TREATMENT: LONGER ACTION AND FEWER SIDE EFFECTS

In the 1960s, it was found that beta-receptors in the lungs differed from those in the heart and **selective** beta-agonists, which worked especially on airways, were introduced. These drugs also lasted much longer and worked very well by inhaler. Such drugs include salbutamol (Ventolin), fenoterol

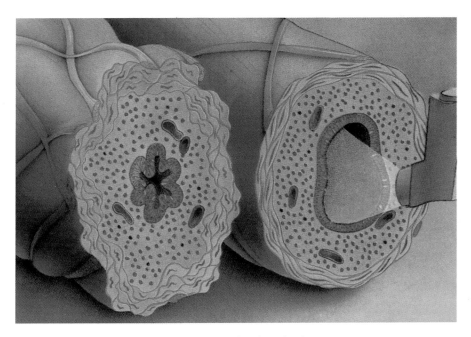

A bronchodilator spray widens the narrowed asthmatic airway.

(Berotec) and terbutaline (Bricanyl), which are the most widely used bronchodilators for asthma. Several similar selective beta-agonists have been developed, but these have no clear advantage over salbutamol or terbutaline. In the past 5 years, new bronchodilators with a 12-hour action have been developed (formoterol, salmeterol). Salmeterol is now available in Britain and several other countries.

HOW DO THEY WORK?

Beta-agonists work mainly in reversing the spasm of airway smooth muscle but may also work to control release of constrictor chemicals from mast cells (see *Chapter 5*). These are therefore good bronchodilators and work extremely well by inhaler. Beta-agonists may last for up to 6 hours (12 hours or more for the new ones like Salmeterol), but don't last as long when the asthma is not well controlled. These drugs are usually inhaled but can also be given as a dry powder or by nebulizer (especially for severe asthma attacks in hospital). They can be taken in tablet form, and long-lasting tablets are now available that may prevent asthma at night. Beta-agonists, as well as relieving wheezing, can also block it from starting. If 2 to 4 puffs of a beta-agonist are taken before exercise or exposure to cold air, then the development of wheezing can usually be blocked for up to 2 hours.

One fact about beta-agonists that is important to recognize is that they do not reduce the inflammation of asthma. They relieve symptoms quickly, so are popular with patients, but do not reverse the inflammation of the airways, which **underlies** asthma. Patients are therefore deceived into thinking that their asthma is better, but the inflammation is masked. What they need, in addition to "when needed" beta-agonists, is an anti-inflammatory treatment taken regularly. Treating asthma with bronchodilators only is like treating appendicitis with pain relievers alone rather than removing the inflamed appendix.

SIDE EFFECTS

When given by inhaler, beta-agonists (relievers) have almost no side effects and are very safe to use. They do not lose their effect if used regularly and there is no question of "addiction" developing. The most common side effect is a feeling of shakiness (because of an effect of the drug on the muscles in the body), and sometimes a pounding, rapid heartbeat, because like adrenaline, the "fight or flight" hormone, they may increase the rate and force of heart beating. These side effects are more common and much more noticeable with the tablet form, but tend to get better when the drug is taken over a long time. Beta-agonists given by inhaler are very safe to use and, even in high doses, do not have serious side effects. However, if you need to use relievers more than once or twice a day to control your asthma, then you need more of the anti-inflammatory (preventer) kind of drug. This is because **"overuse"** of **reliever** inhalers means that your asthma is **out of control as a result of inflammation** of the airway lining. Recent studies have suggested that using these beta-agonists can actually make asthma worse!

2. THEOPHYLLINE

Dr Hyde Salter, a London physician during the last century, noted the value of strong coffee in asthma. Caffeine is the active ingredient and is related to theophylline, which was introduced for relieving attacks of asthma in the 1930s. Theophylline is still a popular treatment although its main disadvantage is the side effects it produces. Theophylline cannot be given by inhaler, so it must be taken in tablet form. (Suppositories were also popular at one time, but they cause irritation of the rectum and are not reliably absorbed into the body). Theophylline is a bronchodilator (reliever), but it is still not known exactly how it works. It has no effect on the inflammation. It is not as good a bronchodilator as the adrenaline-like beta-agonists, however, and, when combined with them, offers little additional benefit to most people. The advantage of theophylline is that long-acting tablet forms are available, some of which last for the whole day. These are particularly useful when taken in the evening for preventing night-time asthma, but should not be needed at all if effective overall asthma control has been achieved by means of the anti-inflammatory (preventer) medicines.

SIDE EFFECTS

The main problem with theophylline is the unwanted effects that may occur at the doses needed to help asthma. The most common side effects are feelings of nausea (sometimes accompanied by vomiting), indigestion, tremulousness, an anxious feeling (like having drunk too much coffee), and headache. More serious side effects are irregular heartbeat and, at very high doses, epileptic seizures. Some people are more susceptible to these side effects, whereas others have little difficulty. Side effects are usually related to the blood level of the drug. If you develop side effects, your doctor will usually take a blood test to measure the level. It may then be necessary to reduce the dose until the best blood level is obtained. The dose needed to give this blood level varies from patient to patient, because it is affected by several factors, such as smoking, age, and often other treatments you may be taking. Because of these problems, theophylline is the second or third choice as a bronchodilator compared with beta-agonists but is sometimes added to beta-agonists to improve asthma control. Nowadays it is used much less than before because better medicines are available for **controlling** asthma rather than simply relieving attacks.

3. ANTICHOLINERGICS

The leaves of the plant *Datura* were smoked in India centuries ago as an asthma treatment. The active ingredient is an anticholinergic and is similar to one contained in Potter's powder, which was smoked as an anti-asthma treatment in the last century. The best known anticholinergic is atropine, derived from the deadly nightshade plant, *Atropa belladona*. These compounds all work by blocking the effects of certain nerves (cholinergic nerves, thus the name of this drug group), which cause narrowing of the air passages by producing contraction of airway muscle. Anticholinergics, sometimes referred to as antimuscarinics, are useful for some patients with asthma where the effects of these nerves contribute to the bronchospasm. But, because the bronchospasm is usually caused by other things as well (such as histamine), these drugs are not usually as good for treating asthma as beta-agonists (which can reverse wheezing, whatever its cause) There are two anticholinergics in common use, ipratropium bromide (Atrovent) which can be given by inhaler or nebulizer, and oxitropium bromide (Oxivent) which is given by metered dose inhaler. These are used as additional bronchodilators in some patients (usually more elderly asthmatics) and, if successful, they have a long-lasting effect – up to 8 hours for Atrovent, and longer for Oxivent. Fortunately they have almost no side effects (occasionally a dry mouth when large doses are given). If you have glaucoma you must avoid getting any of the spray in your eyes. A spacer device attached to the metered dose inhaler (see *Chapter 13*) will assure that the medication goes only into your lungs.

WHICH BRONCHODILATOR?

Of the three types of bronchodilator that are now available for treating asthma, there is no doubt that beta-agonists are best – these produce the greatest effect with the least side effects and work in almost everyone. Most available selective beta-agonists work for about the same length of time (3 to 4 hours), but new beta-agonists have now been developed that last for over 12 hours.

Theophylline is not as good a bronchodilator and may have troublesome side effects. However, it may be a useful additional bronchodilator to add to beta-agonist inhalers in some patients.

Anticholinergics, which are very effective in chronic bronchitis, are the weakest bronchodilators for treating asthma. However, these do have an effect in some asthmatics. They are a second or third choice bronchodilator.

All the bronchodilators (relievers) give relief of asthma symptoms but none have effects against the underlying inflammation that actually **causes** the asthmatic complaints.

ANTI-INFLAMMATORY DRUGS – ASTHMA PREVENTERS AND CONTROLLERS

Since inflammation underlies asthma, it seems logical that treatments that reduce the inflammation should be the most useful in asthma. By controlling the inflammation, the need for bronchodilator drugs will be less, since symptoms will be less common. Indeed, the main aim of asthma control is to use preventer medicines in adequate doses so that the relievers will rarely be needed. Doctors have recently recognized the importance of emphasizing this approach to controlling the disease and are introducing this type of treatment at an earlier stage in asthma. There are two main treatments in this category — steroids and sodium cromoglycate and the related treatment nedocromil sodium.

STEROIDS

Steroids are undoubtedly the most effective anti-asthma treatment now available, but they are still greatly underused. One of the reasons they are not used enough is because patients (and some doctors) are afraid of steroids, having read horror stories about their side effects and their abuse by Olympic athletes. Steroid *tablets* do produce potentially serious unwanted effects when given in a *high dose* over a *long period* (many months or years), but this does **not** apply to steroids given by *inhaler* or to intravenous or oral steroids used for up to a few weeks at a time for controlling asthma flare-ups.

HOW DO THEY WORK?

Although it is not known precisely how steroids work in asthma, it is known that they are particularly effective in **suppressing the asthmatic inflammation**. They are very active against eosinophils, which may be one of the culprits in causing asthma. Reducing the inflammation results in a reduced twitchiness of the airways. Unlike the relievers that act within minutes, steroids take a few hours to have an effect, however, which is important when considering their use in asthma.

STEROID INHALERS

Steroid inhalers, available for the past 20 years, have been a great advance in asthma treatment since steroids can be breathed directly into the airways so that only a small dose is needed. As a rule, not enough steroid is absorbed to have any worrisome effects on the body, so the side effects traditionally associated with steroids do not occur. Steroid inhalers include beclomethasone (Becotide/Becloforte, budesonide (Pulmicort)) and fluticasone (Flixotide). Inhaled steroids need to be taken **regularly** to obtain and maintain control of the asthma. While they begin to take effect in a few days, they may take several weeks to have their maximum effect (because all the inflammation has to be cleaned up and the airways healed). Since these are "preventers" and are not designed to produce immediate relief of symptoms like the bronchodilators (relievers), many people, at first, think they do not work. Inhaled steroids can usually be taken in the morning and in the evening and should be used regularly, for example, before brushing your teeth, as a reminder and to ensure washing the excess from your mouth. Regular use of inhaled steroids usually reduces, and may almost eliminate, the need for bronchodilator inhalers and will reduce or prevent symptoms of asthma (such as exercise asthma, asthma at night, etc.).

SIDE EFFECTS

Side effects are not common. Sometimes a sore mouth and throat develops because of a mould infection in the mouth and throat — recognized by white spots inside the mouth. This can be easily treated with special drug solutions or lozenges. Occasionally the voice becomes husky. These complications are because of the effect of the inhaled steroid in the mouth and throat and can be greatly reduced by the use of a spacer, which reduces the amount of steroids deposited in the mouth (see *Chapter 13*). Rinsing the mouth out with water immediately after inhaling the drug may also help. Additional, relatively uncommon, side effects with very high-dose inhaled steroids (over

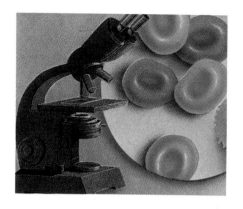

2 g per day beclomethasone or equivalent) include easy bruising, thinning of the skin, and some thinning of bones.

STEROID TABLETS

If asthma is severe or seems to be getting worse in spite of maximum doses of inhaled steroid, it is frequently necessary to take steroid tablets to get or keep it under control. The main problem with long-term use is side effects, and so the lowest dose that controls the asthma should be used. Side effects are minimized by taking the steroid tablets all together in the morning after breakfast (which coincides with the body's production of steroids). The steroid most commonly used is prednisolone.

Steroid tablets or injections are sometimes used every day or every other day in severe asthma and after other medications have been given in maximum doses. The lowest effective dose must be used. This dose may vary according to how severe the asthma is. When the asthma is worse and no longer adequately controlled by the inhaled preventer medicines, higher doses of steroid tablets must be given for a time (usually 1 to 2 weeks), and then tapered off again to the lowest possible dose. Steroid tablets are also given in short courses of 1 to 2 weeks

when the asthma is severe, such as with an infection. Usually you start with 30 to 50 mg (six to ten, 5 mg-tablets) daily and then reduce the dose every day or two to zero. Alternatively, six tablets may be taken every day for 1 to 2 weeks and then stopped (or the previous maintenance dose, if any, resumed).

SIDE EFFECTS OF STEROID TABLETS OR INJECTIONS

Side effects, which occur only after long-term use, may be serious and disfiguring, include increase in weight due to overeating and retention of water, a swollen looking moonface, excess hair, thinning of the bones (which makes broken bones more likely), thinning and bruising of the skin, an increase in blood pressure, and occasionally cataracts. In children, steroids cause stunting of growth (see *Chapter 14*). High doses may expose a previous tendency to develop diabetes. Very rarely, the hip joint may be destroyed due to loss of blood supply.

Steroids at a dose of 10 mg (2 tablets) daily or more for a long time suppress the body's own production of steroids, which are needed to respond to stress (such as a surgical operation or major accident). If steroids are stopped abruptly, after they have been taken for many weeks, months or years, then the body may not be able to respond properly to these stresses, which means that low blood pressure and a state of shock develop. It is therefore important that you carry a card or bracelet saying that you are on regular steroid tablets, so that a doctor will be alerted to give you replacement steroids if an emergency arises. This is not necessary if you are using the usual dose of inhaled steroids but may be needed if total body doses of inhaled steroids of over 1.5 to 2 mg daily are being taken. This small inhaled dose has a beneficial effect on the lungs

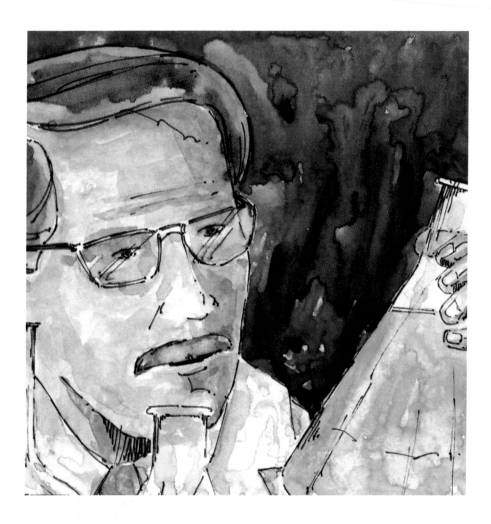

similar to 30 or 40 mg of steroid tablets but an effect on the body of only about 5 mg daily of steroid taken by mouth. Using a metered dose inhaler (MDI) add-on device, which keeps the large drug particles that are not useful for treatment out of the body, further reduces the total body dose from the inhaled steroid by 75 percent, thereby making side effects of little or no concern in most patients (see *Chapter 13*).

CROMOGLYCATE (INTAL)

Cromoglycate (Intal) is an anti-asthma treatment that was originally derived from an Egyptian herbal remedy. It was found to prevent wheezing after exposure to allergic reactions, although it is not a bronchodilator. It works only if given **before** exposure to the allergen. It is still not known exactly how it works, but it was originally believed to work against mast cells (explaining why it gave a good protection against the allergic type of asthma). It now seems likely that it also works against the other cells involved in asthmatic inflammation, including eosinophils.

Cromoglycate is therefore used as a preventer in a similar way to inhaled steroids. It can be taken using a dry powder inhaler (Spinhaler) or by a metered dose inhaler (MDI) taken 2–4 times a day. It is a preventive treatment and reduces the symptoms of asthma with time. It also blocks exercise asthma when taken **before** exercise, but not if taken to relieve asthma after exercise. Cromoglycate has virtually no side effects and, for this reason, is the preferred anti-inflammatory treatment for children with mild to moderate asthma.

Cromoglycate is not as effective as steroids and does not work on every patient. Although cromoglycate is often used in children, inhaled steroids are the most effective and economical anti-inflammatory drugs and are our first choice in all age groups.

NEDOCROMIL (TILADE)

This is a new cromoglycate-like medication that is similar to cromoglycate in effectiveness and in the way it works. A mint-flavoured inhaler is now available because some patients complained about a bitter taste.

KETOTIFEN

Ketotifen (Zaditen), a type of antihistamine (see below), is a treatment that may benefit some children with very mild asthma. It may be taken by mouth, which makes it easy to use but it may take several weeks or months to show any benefit. Drowsiness is a side effect, although less so in children. However, ketotifen is much less effective than inhaled steroids or even cromoglycate.

OTHER TREATMENTS

DESENSITIZING INJECTIONS

A course of injections to reduce allergic reactions is popular in the United States and some continental European countries, but less so in the United Kingdom, Canada and Australia. Patients are injected with very dilute solutions of allergen, and the strength of injections is increased at regular intervals. The principle of this course of injections is that the body will be stimulated to produce blocking factors, which will block the allergic response. While there has been some success in treating hay fever with injections of grass pollen extract, there is not much evidence that allergy injections are helpful in asthma. This may be partly because a number of different allergens are usually involved, and it would be necessary to desensitize against each one. The course of injections is expensive and time-consuming for the patient, and it is not certain how long any benefit lasts. The major disadvantage of allergy injections is their potential danger. Mild reactions to the injections, such as swelling at the site of injection, are common, but severe reactions occasionally occur—these are a form of allergic shock that can very occasionally be fatal. Several deaths were recently reported in Sweden, and the Committee on Safety of Medicines in the United Kingdom issued a strongly worded letter advising all doctors against using allergy injections. Thus, allergy injections cannot be recommended in asthma, since they have no proven effect and they are potentially dangerous. Some doctors believe allergy injections should be continued for many years, but there is little scientific evidence that, even for hay fever, more than 2 or 3 years of treatment is of use in most people.

ANTIHISTAMINES

Antihistamine drugs, such as promethazine (Phenergan), chlorpheniramine (Piriton), and triprolidine (Pro-actidil), block the effects of histamine and are useful in treating hay fever and allergic nose diseases. The problem with the original antihistamines is that they cause drowsiness and should not be taken when driving or working at jobs that require you to be alert. Recently, a new generation of long-acting antihistamines that do not cause sedation have been developed, such as terfenadine (Triludan), astemizole (Hismanal), and loratadine (Claritin). These can also be given in higher doses because they do not cause drowsiness. However, even these new antihistamines are not useful in treating asthma (the reason being that chemical mediators other than histamine are also involved).

ANTIBIOTICS

Antibiotics, such as penicillin, erythromycin, amoxicillin, and co-trimoxazole (Septrin), are helpful for chest infections caused by bacteria (severe bronchitis or pneumonia), but bacterial infections are not often the cause of asthma attacks (which are usually a result of viruses or virus-like germs when infection is involved). Antibiotics are commonly given for an asthma attack but are only rarely needed (since virus infections do not respond). The phlegm may become yellow or greenish during an asthma attack, but even this does not mean that there is a chest infection, since the increased number of eosinophils (see *Chapter 5*) in phlegm during an asthma attack gives this appearance.

11 Controlling Asthma and Treating Attacks: A Logical Approach

As you have learned so far from the preceding chapters, asthma is an inflammatory condition of the airways. Its basic cause is not yet completely understood, but because excellent anti-inflammatory medications have become available during the past 20 years, most people with asthma can achieve excellent control of the condition and lead almost completely normal lives. Unfortunately, some asthmatics have such severe inflammation of their air passages or some permanent narrowing, because of poor asthma control over many years or because of smoking, that they cannot be returned to normal, even when anti-inflammatory medications are used in the largest possible doses or even if several medications are used in combination. In such cases the aim should be to achieve and maintain the best possible result.

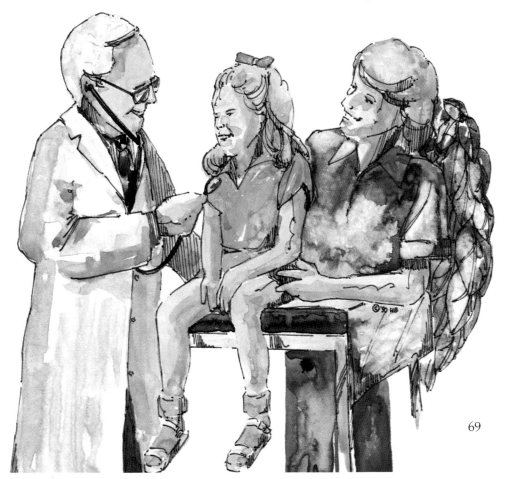

AIMS OF TREATMENT

The main aims of treatment are:

1. Eliminate all identifiable causes of asthma to "cure" the condition (see *Chapters 8* and *10*).
2. Achieve and maintain control of asthma with medications if a specific cause cannot be found and eliminated.
3. Prevent severe flare-ups by treating deterioration vigorously and early as described later in this chapter.

HOW TO TELL IF ASTHMA IS UNDER CONTROL

Your asthma should be under control under the following conditions:

1. You should be virtually free of symptoms such as coughing, wheezing, breathlessness, chest tightness, or phlegm production almost all the time.
2. If symptoms do occur, they should be mild, infrequent, and readily relieved by your bronchodilator (reliever) inhaler, which should be effective for at least 4 hours (over 12 hours with the long-acting bronchodilator aerosols that are becoming available). If you need the short-acting bronchodilator aerosols more than once or twice a day, control is not ideal.
3. Normal activities of daily living, including work or school, should not be interfered with, and you should be able to exercise, even strenuously and in cold weather. You should not have to miss sleep, work, or play.
4. You should **never** (or almost never) need to be hospitalized because of asthma.
5. Your medicines should **never** (or almost never) cause troublesome side effects.
6. The airflow rates measured by your doctor or by you (if you have a peak flow meter at home) should be normal or near normal at rest. If they are somewhat reduced, they should certainly return to normal or near normal shortly after you have used your bronchodilator (reliever) inhaler. The peak flow readings should not vary more than 10 to 15 percent from morning to night. The morning value is usually the lower one.

When your doctor begins to treat your asthma, the initial treatment will usually be particularly vigorous (often using larger doses of the medicines than will later be required to keep you under control). This is to see if your

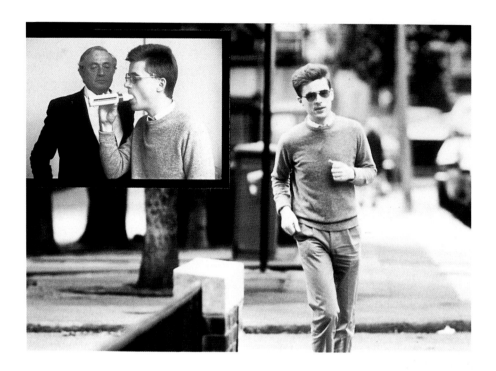

symptoms can be brought under excellent control and also to make sure that the flow rates return to normal or near normal.

PRINCIPLES OF TREATMENT

1. Treatment must keep you normal or at the best possible level.
2. **Avoiding** the things that may injure your airways and cause inflammation is better than treatment with medications. For example, some asthmatics find that they need little or no medication if they get rid of the cat to which they have become allergic, change the job that has caused occupational asthma (see *Chapter 16*), or stop smoking. The medication you may be taking to control other conditions should also be carefully reviewed with your doctor, because asthma may be made worse by **aspirin**, and most arthritis medicines (in about one percent of asthmatics), some heart medications (**beta-blockers**), and eye drops used to treat glaucoma (**beta-blockers**). (**Note**: Asthmatics should never take beta-blockers. These drugs may cause severe and life-threatening attacks or even death.)

3. Controlling the underlying inflammation that causes the airway spasm is much better than simply treating the spasm itself. Controlling the inflammation is best accomplished by avoiding potentially harmful factors (see *Chapters 8 and 10*). If this is not sufficient to achieve control, inhaled steroid (or sometimes cromoglycate [Intal]) or steroid tablets (during asthma flare-ups and for control of the most severe forms of asthma) can be used.

4. Neither bronchodilator inhalers nor theophylline tablets treat the underlying inflammation and so are not effective in reducing the **severity** of the disease.

71

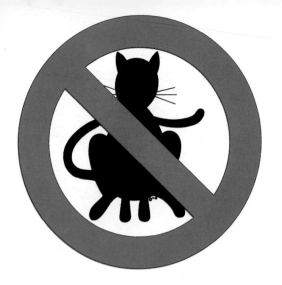

5. The proper assessment and treatment of asthma include the following:
   a) Making the diagnosis.
   b) Providing vigorous treatment after the diagnosis has been made in order to establish control quickly by avoiding, if possible, the things that have caused the problem and by the use of medications.
   c) Over the next few weeks or months, you and your doctor can establish what medications are needed and the lowest possible dose that will keep your asthma under control or maintain the best possible result.
   d) You and your doctor should develop a written "action plan," to be reviewed with you until you completely understand it, so that flare-ups can be treated early before they become serious enough to interfere with your normal activities or even require visits to the hospital emergency room or admission to hospital.
   e) For achieving and maintaining good control of the asthma, your cooperation in starting treatment of asthma deterioration is essential. Thus, the better you understand the disease, learn to recognize the early features of deterioration, and learn to take early corrective action, the better you will be able to maintain control and lead a normal life. This book, as well as pamphlets that your doctor, allergy or asthma association, or support group may provide, should greatly help you with this.
   f) After the asthma is first diagnosed and treatment has been started, you and your doctor should meet regularly, depending on how severe the problem is and how well the initial treatment seems to be working. Many GPs now hold regular asthma clinics in their practice which are run by a specially trained asthma nurse.
   g) If the asthma is particularly severe and/or does not respond to an appropriate treatment programme within a reasonable period of time, it may be necessary for your doctor to send you to other doctors who are specialists in treating lung disease and/or allergies. These specialists may suggest readjusting your medications, using larger doses,

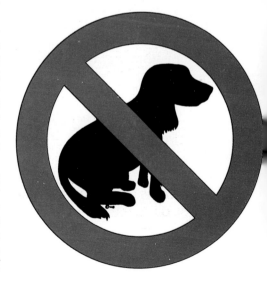

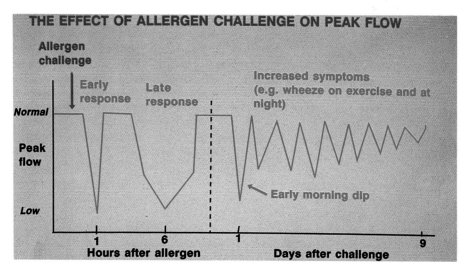

THE EFFECT OF ALLERGEN CHALLENGE ON PEAK FLOW

Allergen challenge

Early response

Late response

Increased symptoms (e.g. wheeze on exercise and at night)

Normal

Peak flow

Low

Early morning dip

1   6   1   9
Hours after allergen   Days after challenge

or sometimes, with your complete understanding and approval, even trying new and experimental medications. Thus you may also be asked to volunteer for a research study with a new medication that may later turn out to become one of the standard treatments.

TREATMENT PLAN

After your doctor has established the diagnosis by asking you questions about your illness and examining you, you may have a chest X-ray, a series of allergy skin tests, breathing tests before and after taking two puffs from the bronchodilator inhaler, and perhaps asthma provocation tests. You may also receive on loan, or be advised to purchase, a peak flow meter, so that you can record the peak flow at least twice a day at home. This gives your doctor information about the severity of the asthma (all of these tests are described in *Chapter 9*).

ASTHMA TREATMENT TO ESTABLISH CONTROL OR ACHIEVE THE BEST RESULT

First and foremost, you should do everything you can to eliminate poss-

ible underlying causes of the asthma (see *Chapter 8*). If you have sinus infections or indigestion, these factors could also contribute to the asthma and should be discussed with your doctor. Avoiding potentially harmful factors is very important, because these may cause or increase the inflammation of the airway, thus leading to increased symptoms. They may even trigger sudden, very severe and potentially life-threatening episodes of asthma.

Once it has been established what factors in your environment may be causing or contributing to the asthma, your doctor will give you detailed information about avoidance (see pages 146–149). In general, avoidance procedures should be practical and should take account of observations you have made about things that affect you. If possible, you should not undertake excessive or unnecessary avoidance procedures that may make life particularly difficult, unless these have been shown to be especially useful. When in doubt, avoidance procedures should always be discussed with your doctor to make sure that they are appropriate (see instructions about avoiding allergies to food colourings

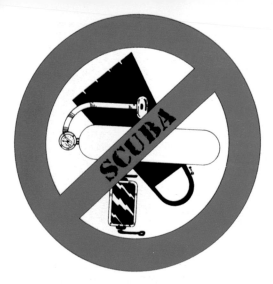

and food preservatives; see page 146).

Allergen injection treatments have been suggested as a preventative asthma treatment, but these have not been found particularly useful in most asthmatics (see *Chapter 10*).

While exercise may cause transient asthma attacks when the asthma is not under good control, avoiding exercise should not be part of the treatment of well-controlled asthma. Indeed, the ability to exercise more or less normally (once a good state of physical fitness has been achieved) is one of the important features of well-controlled asthma. An important exception is scuba diving. Asthmatics should **not** engage in this activity because a small mucus plug could lead to overdistension of air sacs in the lung during the ascent. The result could be life threatening, because the lungs may collapse or air bubbles may enter the blood and so move to the brain, causing a stroke. Thus, reputable scuba training programs will not accept asthmatics.

If it is impossible for you to completely avoid allergens (for instance, you are going to a friend's house where there are cats or dogs to which you are allergic), you may prevent or greatly reduce the severity of an asthma attack or nose blockage due to rhinitis by using cromoglycate. This should be inhaled into your lungs and nose 10 or 15 minutes before exposure, and the medication continued for a few days until all the symptoms have cleared (see *Chapter 10*). Increasing the dose of the inhaled steroid (usually by doubling the amount that keeps you under control most of the time) usually corrects the post-exposure asthma flare-up and shortens the time until control is again established. Extra puffs of inhaled steroid 10 or 15 minutes before exposure (unlike cromoglycate) will **not** assist in preventing the reaction at the time of exposure.

CONTROLLING ASTHMA WITH MEDICATIONS

If avoidance procedures are successful, these will probably prevent future episodes of asthma and may even allow control of the condition without medications. However, this is usually the case only if there is allergy to one or two easily avoided things (like domestic pets or shellfish).

Medications are required:
1. To bring and keep current asthma under good control,
2. To treat flare-ups of asthma that are a result of allergy-causing substances, and
3. To relieve attacks related to exercise or cold air exposure.

Inhaled medications are preferred because they are very effective in low doses and cause few, if any, side effects.

The amount of treatment required when your doctor first sees you will depend on how severe your asthma is at the time, as well as on the type and dosage of the medicines that you are already taking. If the asthma is not severe, the aim of treatment will be to bring your asthma under control or to achieve the best possible result within 1 or 2 weeks. The severity of your

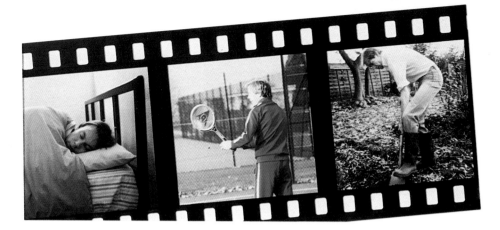

asthma can be judged by your doctor based on the symptoms, the flow rate measurements, and the number of times per day you need to use the bronchodilator inhaler to stay reasonably free of symptoms.

It is convenient for the sake of deciding how much treatment is required **at any given time** to divide the severity of asthma into four levels, as follows:

Severity Level 1 – The asthma is well controlled as outlined previously (see page 70, "How to Tell if Asthma Is Under Control"). Bronchodilators are needed once a day or less.

Severity Level 2 – Symptoms are present from time to time on most days and bronchodilator (reliever) inhalers are required two or more times daily. If you measure the peak flow rate at home with a peak flow meter, the results are 15 to 20 percent below the predicted or best achievable values. Peak flow is 20 to 30 percent lower in the morning than in the evening.

Severity Level 3 – Symptoms of breathlessness and chest tightness occur frequently, interfere with sleep, or occur first thing in the morning when you wake up, and the bronchodilator inhaler is needed more than three or four times a day. The peak flow reading is 20 to 40 percent below the predicted value or the best result that was previously achieved, and the variability

from morning to night is more than 30 percent below normal or the best achievable values.

Severity Level 4 – Asthma symptoms are present at rest and are not returned to normal by bronchodilator inhalers. The peak flow reading is more than 40 percent below your normal or best achievable value.

In some asthmatics, the symptoms are the best guide to deterioration (along with the number of times per day the bronchodilator inhaler is needed), while in others the airway narrowing becomes severe before they realize they are in trouble. If you are an asthmatic who is sensitive to changes in your symptoms, adjustments in medication are best related to symptoms and the need for increased bronchodilator puffs. If you are an asthmatic who does not readily perceive deterioration early, it is essential that you carefully measure peak flows every day so you can adjust the level of treatment according to the severity level. Following these instructions will assist you to avoid serious attacks by intervening early.

TREATING ASTHMA ACCORDING TO SEVERITY LEVELS

TREATING SEVERITY LEVEL 1

If the asthma is extremely mild and infrequent, with symptoms occurring no more than once or twice a week,

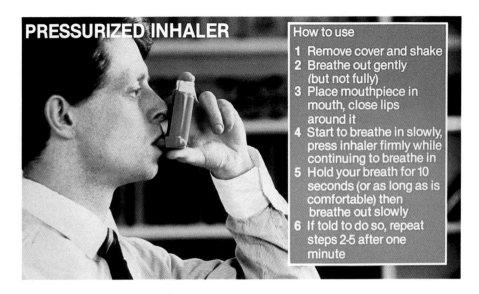

usually on exercise or exposure to cold air, then bronchodilator inhalers alone are probably all that is needed. However, many asthmatics tend to have symptoms on a more or less regular basis, and thus do not fall into this category. Symptoms may vary in severity, but are generally mild and there may be long periods of relative freedom from symptoms between episodes, during which symptoms are absent for several weeks or months. At this level, cromoglycate as well as the bronchodilator (reliever) inhaler may be needed before exercise to control symptoms on exercise or cold air exposure if the **bronchodilator alone** is not effective in a dose of 2–4 puffs taken 5–10 minutes beforehand.

TREATING SEVERITY LEVEL 2

At this severity level, symptoms occur frequently—up to several times a day—although they are usually mild to moderate and rarely interfere with sleep. The treatment at this level consists of an anti-inflammatory preventer medication such as daily inhaled steroid, usually from one of the low-dose per puff (50 μg beclomethasone or equivalent) steroid inhalers (see *Chapter 10*), starting with four puffs twice a day, along with a bronchodilator inhaler as needed. You know that good control has been achieved with this medication if after 7 to 10 days the need for bronchodilator puffs has decreased to once or twice daily. By this time peak flow rates should be near normal (or the best achievable) and variability of peak flow from morning to night (diurnal variation) should be small (less than 15 percent). If this has not occurred, then a larger dose of the inhaled steroid is needed.

At this level of severity, cromoglycate may sometimes be almost as effective as low dose inhaled steroids. Some doctors prefer to start with this drug, particularly in children. The starting dose is usually two puffs inhaled four times a day, although twice this dose may be required as preventative medication in some asthmatics. If cromoglycate does not work very well, it should be replaced by low dose inhaled steroids (for example, four 50-μg puffs 200 μg twice a day of beclomethasone or equivalent).

TREATING SEVERITY LEVEL 3

At this severity level, symptoms of asthma are present most of the time prior to treatment and cause awakening at night, early morning chest tightness, and the need to use the bronchodilator inhaler four or more times a day. This indicates the need for higher doses of inhaled steroid up to a total daily dose of 1 to 2 mg (rarely, even more), usually taken morning and night (for convenience). With more severe asthma, however, the same total number of puffs may work better if given 3 or 4 times a day. When inhaled steroids are used, metered dose inhaler spacer devices (as described in *Chapter 13*) should be used, particularly with the larger doses often needed to control level 3 severity asthma. If maximum doses of the inhaled steroid have been used and control is still less than ideal, some of the other medications described in *Chapter 10* can be tried to "fine tune" the treatment and to try to avoid the need to take steroid tablets regularly. At this point, careful trials of adding one of the theophylline drugs or even an anticholinergic inhaler might be helpful. If not, then it is necessary to go on to severity level 4 treatment, which means adding cortisone (tablets prednisolone) as long-term treatment. At this severity level it is probably a good idea to consult an asthma specialist on at least one occasion to be sure that you are obtaining as much help as possible. Repeat visits to the specialist every year or two will assure that you get the benefit of new developments as soon as they become available.

TREATING SEVERE ASTHMA

Treating asthma of this severity almost *always requires the help of a specialist* to bring and keep the asthma under control. The treatment consists of maximum doses of inhaled steroids (up to 3 mg of beclomethasone, budesonide, or equivalent per day) administered in a dose of 500–1000 μg four times a day by means of a holding chamber type of metered dose inhaler accessory device to reduce the side effects to a minimum. In addition, inhaled beta-agonists (adrenaline-like bronchodilators, 2 to 4 puffs up to six times daily) almost always are needed. A long acting beta-agonist should always be tried (salmeterol 1–2 puffs twice a day). Theophylline tablets and/or an anticholinergic aerosol may be helpful, and this should be established with the help of your doctor by carefully monitored trials of treatment.

If the asthma remains poorly controlled (symptoms at rest, on exercise, waking from sleep, asthma attacks, poor response to bronchodilator inhalers, which are required more than 4 to 6 times a day), prednisolone tablets are needed in doses sufficient to control the asthma. Repeated attempts must be made, at the frequent follow-up visits, to reduce the prednisolone to the lowest possible dose. If control of the asthma allows, the prednisolone tablets should be given on alternate days to reduce cortisone-related side effects to a minimum.

In some patients with the most severe and uncontrollable asthma, attempts have been made to improve control and reduce the dose of prednisolone by using immunosuppressive drugs (e.g., methotrexate) in small doses. Gold injections (like those given to people with rheumatoid arthritis) have also been tried. These have had some success in pilot research studies. Such medications may unfortunately have potentially serious side effects and must be used cautiously, only in situations where the usual treatments have not been very effective and high doses of prednisolone are needed on a long-term basis.

Before proceeding to the addition of cortisone tablets, you and your doctor should carefully review the diagnosis of asthma and all of the current treatment to make sure that no other conditions are making it difficult to control your asthma (see *Chapters 7 and 15*). You and your doctor should also review all of the medications that have been prescribed to be sure that you are taking the appropriate doses and that you are using the aerosol devices properly, so that the medication is really getting into your lungs.

BEGINNING TREATMENT

If your symptoms are bothersome at the time you first see the doctor, you will often be given a short course of prednisolone tablets to bring the asthma under rapid control (e.g., 50 mg of prednisolone daily for 1 week or occasionally longer, followed by 25 mg daily for a second week). Similar courses of prednisolone may be used for future flare-ups of asthma if **increasing** the dose of the **inhaled steroid** (usually to twice what was needed for maintenance) when the asthma **begins to get worse** does not bring the problem under control.

Once you have achieved good control, frequent follow-up (every 2 to 6 weeks) with your doctor may be needed at first to make sure that things are going well, to answer questions you may have, and to adjust the treatment levels to **the lowest dose that will keep you well** controlled and in severity level 1 if possible.

Antihistamines, which may be useful for treating allergic rhinitis, are **of little or no value** for treating asthma.

CONTINUING TREATMENT

Once you and your doctor have established the ideal level of treatment for you, repeat visits can be stretched out to many weeks or months. Finally, with really good control of the asthma, annual visits are probably all that is needed, unless the asthma slips out of control and does not improve to your previous best levels after you increase the dose of preventer (anti-inflammatory) aerosol inhaler as indicated above and according to your doctor's specific instructions. You will, of course, also contact your doctor at once if the asthma seems to be getting worse rapidly; if peak flow readings remain reduced by 15 percent or more below normal or the previous best values for more than 24 to 48 hours; or if, having been at severity level 1, you move to severity level 3 or 4 in spite of attempts to correct deterioration by doubling the inhaled steroid puffs after you have slipped from severity level 1 to severity level 2.

If you have been under good control for many months at a given level of treatment, then you can discuss with your doctor the possibility of reducing the level of one or more of your medications or even discontinuing medications that may no longer be required. Drugs that can be decreased or perhaps eliminated are usually the bronchodilator tablets (particularly theophylline), while the anti-inflammatory drugs (such as inhaled steroids or cromoglycate) are usually continued for long periods of time, often indefinitely. An important exception to this is people with well-defined allergic asthma, who may only require continuous treatment during the allergy season and for a relatively short time afterwards. Many people with asthma are advised to take severity level 2 or 3 medication just before the beginning of the allergy season that they know from past experience will cause them difficulty, and then gradually taper the medication off over about 4 weeks after the allergy season has ended.

Maintaining constant good control of your asthma is **all-important** for preventing severe and potentially life-threatening attacks. Also, regular treatment may, over many months, actually produce a fundamental improvement in the disease and lead to a decrease in your need for as much inhaled steroid (preventer) medications with time. Finally, since there is increasing evidence that the ongoing inflammation associated with poorly controlled asthma may, over many years, lead to permanent damage to the airways, keeping the asthma under control will probably prevent this permanent injury to your lungs.

NOTE: Never discontinue your preventer medication without your doctor's specific instructions to do so!

How to Treat Asthma Flare-ups

Following the treatment plan outlined above will keep your asthma under control most of the time. However, episodes of deterioration may still occur if you are exposed to agents that may injure the airways such as allergens, chemicals in the air at your job or food preservatives to which you may be sensitive, and infections, particularly those caused by viruses like the influenza virus.

When these asthma flare-ups occur, you will **always** need more treatment to bring them under control. For this purpose, you should have an action plan that you have worked out with your doctor to prevent deterioration and restore control.

Action Plan for Early Treatment of Asthma Flare-ups

If your asthma symptoms are under control (i.e., virtually no symptoms) or at the best possible level as a result of close collaboration between you and your doctor, and if you have established your maintenance treatment level and normal or best possible peak flow rate, this will be the basis for deciding whether additional treatment is needed in the future.

When to Start the Action Plan

Starting the action plan can be based on

- Increased asthma symptoms; for example, more breathlessness on exertion that previously could be done with ease, chest tightness on getting up in the morning, waking up at night with asthma, onset of cough.
- The need for increased bronchodilator puffs (previously you were using the bronchodilator [reliever] inhaler only once or twice a day, but you now require it three or four times daily), or
- A decrease in the peak flow (more than 15 to 20 percent below normal or the previous best possible values) that you were able to achieve following use of your bronchodilator inhaler on the maintenance treatment programme.

The Action Plan in Action (A Recipe for Successful Treatment of Most Asthma Attacks)

An example of a typical action plan to quickly relieve an asthma attack is as follows: (Note that this assumes you are already taking relievers (bronchodilators) and preventers (inhaled steroids or cromoglycate) and have previously been well controlled.)

To relieve the breathlessness quickly:
1. If two puffs from the bronchodilator inhaler have not been effective (assuming that two puffs usually are), take four more puffs of the bronchodilator medication—one every 30 seconds. Wait about 5 minutes for a response.
2. If you are still breathless take one additional bronchodilator puff each minute until the breathlessness is relieved or you tremble or notice

palpitations of your heart, whichever comes first. Then stop taking additional puffs, but if necessary, this could be repeated every 20 to 30 minutes for severe asthma.

3. If you have been measuring peak flow rate, you can expect it to improve by about 50 percent (for example, from 250 L/min to 375 L/min). If this works, proceed to section below. If not, then you should contact your doctor or the hospital emergency department at once.

To restore control:

1. Double the preventer medication (e.g., cromoglycate [Intal], inhaled steroids [Becotide, Becloforte, Pulmicort, Flixotide, etc.]), so, if already taking two puffs four times daily, increase to four puffs four times daily. If already taking four puffs four times daily, proceed to 2 (below).

2. If there has not been noticeable improvement after 12 to 24 hours or if you are getting steadily worse, start prednisolone pills, 30 to 50 mg daily (or as suggested by your doctor) for about 1 week or until clearly improved.

3. Discuss with your doctor how rapidly to reduce the prednisolone and what (if any) maintenance dose is needed. The usual treatment is one half of the first week's dose for a second week, after which prednisolone tablets are usually discontinued since most asthmatics do not require on-going treatment with prednisolone if they are taking inhaled steroids (preventers) in sufficient doses. Severe, unstable asthmatics may, however, need long-term prednisolone (taken on alternate days if possible to reduce side effects) along with inhaled steroids in maximum doses to keep the need for prednisolone tablets to an absolute minimum.

ACTION PLAN NOT WORKING?

If the action plan outlined above has not started to work within 6 to 12 hours, if you continue to be breathless while sitting quietly, or if the bronchodilator inhaler works for less than 4 hours, you should immediately contact your doctor or go to the nearest hospital casualty department.

ACTION PLANNING USING PEAK FLOW AS A GUIDE

An action plan can also be based on measurement of the peak flow rate if you regularly use a peak flow meter. For example, if your best peak flow rate is 500 L/min and for 24 hours the peak flow after using the bronchodilator inhaler is less than:

1. 425 (85 percent of the best previous result) — double the dose of inhaled steroid and continue at that level until readings are again within 90 percent of normal or the previous best result.

2. 300 (60 percent of best result) — start prednisolone 50 mg daily until readings are again within 90 percent of the best result (this will usually take 4 to 7 days).

3. 250 (50 percent of best result) — take an additional 50 mg of prednisolone, follow the instructions detailed under Ⓐ (How to relieve breathlessness quickly), and go to the nearest hospital emergency department or to your doctor at once.

BE PREPARED!

In order to be able to follow this action plan, you must keep a supply of prednisolone tablets on hand at all times. You should take these with you when you are away on business or on vacation. You should also have a spare supply of bronchodilator inhalers so that you do not run out in an emergency. Occasionally, on your doctor's advice, you may need to keep on hand automatic injection syringes of adrenaline for injection into your thigh tissue, particularly if your attacks are sudden, severe, and respond poorly to even many puffs of bronchodilator. Such injections are nowadays usually used to treat very severe anaphylactic episodes that are most commonly due to allergic reactions to foods, such as peanuts or shellfish. Bee sting (wasp, hornet) sensitivity may also cause life-threatening reactions. The best "first-aid" treatment for these reactions is adrenaline by auto-injectable syringe or even by inhalation of 10–15 puffs from a Medihaler epi inhaler.

SPECIAL TREATMENT MEASURES

Patients with severe asthma may sometimes need a home nebulizer system to provide bronchodilator medication, but this is **not a substitute** for effective treatment of deterioration with increased doses of inhaled steroids or, if necessary, with steroid tablets, even though temporary relief may be obtained with the nebulizer. Furthermore, nebulizers are now rapidly being replaced by holding chamber devices such as the Nebuhaler® or Volumatic®, which provide reliable delivery of bronchodilator (reliever) puffs from metered dose inhalers, even when the asthma attack is severe (see *Chapter 12*). In rare cases, a home oxygen supply may be needed, particularly for patients who develop sudden severe attacks far from a medical facility that can provide emergency treatment. An oxygen supply may also be needed by asthmatics who have such severe damage to their airways (perhaps as a result of also being cigarette smokers) that the oxygen level in their blood is chronically low, becomes very low during sleep, or falls to very low levels when walking about or exercising.

Oxygen should be used in this way only on the advice of and under the supervision of your doctor.

FOLLOW-UP VISITS

Follow-up visits with your doctor are **extremely important**. When things are going well, such visits can be relatively infrequent, but in any case should occur at least once a year. When things are going less than ideally, you should implement the action plan outlined in this chapter **early on** and arrange to see your doctor as soon as possible!

With time you will become expert at self-care of your asthma over long periods of time and will achieve a large measure of independence from unexpected and frightening asthma attacks. With the information provided, self-care of your asthma should be less difficult for you than self-care of diabetes is for a person with diabetes, but it is just as important.

A medical summary card containing information about your asthma and other medical problems, as well as a list of your medications and a summary of the action plans, is included with this book. We suggest that you ask your doctor to help you fill it out. If it is filled out in pencil it can be changed as your medication is adjusted. If you show it to any doctor that you may visit in the future, it will provide helpful information that will assist in your care.

CHANGING OVER FROM LONG-TERM STEROID TABLET TREATMENT TO AEROSOL STEROIDS: A WORD OF CAUTION

If you are one of the asthmatics whose condition is so severe that you have been taking steroid tablets (prednisolone) for many months or years, it may now be possible to replace all or a large part of the dose of tablets with the much safer inhaled steroid medications. However, taking steroid tablets (or, rarely, injections) for prolonged periods leads to a marked decrease in the production of your own cortisone from the adrenal glands (small structures near the kidneys). Normally, these glands produce the cortisone that we all need every day, and they are also able to greatly increase the amount of cortisone produced if our bodies are placed under conditions of stress such as serious infections, injury in severe accidents, or major surgical procedures.

If you have been taking prednisolone pills for long periods of time, the adrenal glands may lose their ability to produce enough cortisone for your day-to-day needs or to increase the amount of cortisone required to deal with physically stressful situations. The symptoms associated with inadequate cortisone production include widespread aches and pains in your joints, loss of appetite, a feeling of nausea, severe vomiting, and marked weakness and dizziness because of low blood pressure resulting from loss of salt and fluid from your system. Unless the necessary cortisone is replaced, you might even die of lack of this important hormone.

Obviously then, any reduction in the cortisone you have been receiving in tablet form or by injection over many months or years should be undertaken gradually and only under the supervision of your doctor. The steroid pills must be withdrawn at a rate that will allow your own steroid production to resume and provide you with the necessary protection from physical stress. It may take a year or two after reducing the prednisolone pills to very low doses (less than 7.5 mg per day) before your own adrenal glands are producing sufficient cortisone to sustain you under normal conditions. It may take up to 5 years for the glands to be able to respond normally to physically stressful situations by adequately increasing the amount of cortisone they produce.

If you have been taking steroids for more than a few weeks, you should make sure of the following:
1. The dose should be decreased gradually under your doctor's supervision before being discontinued. Your doctor may do a blood test to be sure that the glands are working (Synacthen Test).
2. You should get a bracelet to let doctors know that you were taking steroids on a long-term basis, so that if you should be found unconscious (such as after a car accident), you would immediately be given supplements of the cortisone you need to deal with the injury or any necessary surgery.
3. You must let any new doctors know that you took steroid tablets over long periods of time to alert them to your need to have cortisone supplements for surgery.
4. You should have a supply of prednisolone tablets on hand so that if you develop symptoms of severe asthma or steroid withdrawal such as those outlined above, you can start a dose of steroid tablets (approximately 10 mg of prednisolone daily if you are not particularly ill, 50 mg daily or more, as advised by your doctor, if you have a fever and are sick). You should also contact your doctor at once.

The majority of asthmatics who had to depend on steroid pills before the inhaled steroids became available can now usually stop taking prednisolone tablets if large enough doses of inhaled steroid are used and the prednisolone is withdrawn gradually as above. The result of this change in treatment will

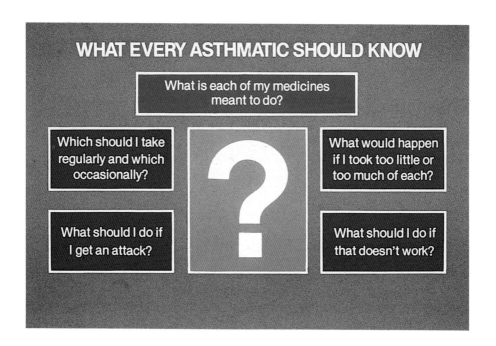

WHAT EVERY ASTHMATIC SHOULD KNOW

What is each of my medicines meant to do?

Which should I take regularly and which occasionally?

What would happen if I took too little or too much of each?

What should I do if I get an attack?

What should I do if that doesn't work?

be that your bloated appearance gradually returns to normal and the risk of the various side effects associated with taking steroid tablets for long periods of time will greatly decrease. Typical side effects include a moon face, a tendency for the bones to be weakened, a predisposition to develop cataracts, and increased susceptibility to infection. Since these effects are related to the dose of the steroid tablets or injections that you need to keep you under control, many of the side effects will be greatly decreased in severity even if you are only able to partially reduce the dose of the cortisone tablets of injections (the so-called "steroid tablet sparing effect" of the inhaled steroids). With the availability of high dose-per-puff inhaled steroid medications (such as budesonide [Pulmicort], 200 μg per puff, beclomethasone [Becloforte], 250 μg per puff, and fluticasone [Flixotide], an experimental high-potency drug, most, even fairly severe, asthmatics should be able to

stop taking steroid tablets completely with time or at least switch to prednisolone tablets every second day (a technique that greatly reduces side effects).

Steroid tablets and injections (but not inhaled steroids) may bring out a tendency to develop diabetes, so that if you are taking blood sugar-lowering medicines, and you reduce or discontinue prednisolone tablets, you will probably need lower doses or insulin or blood sugar-lowering tablets. As the prednisolone is reduced, you may sometimes even be able to stop diabetes treatment completely. Of course, the treatment of your diabetes should only be changed under your doctor's close supervision.

If the blood sugar becomes too low (because insulin or the blood sugar-lowering tablets have not been decreased enough as the steroid tablets are reduced), you may experience spells of weakness, sweating, light-headedness, confusion, or even un-

83

consciousness (doctors call this a hypoglycaemic reaction). During the phase of lightheadedness, sweating, and weakness, taking a few sugar cubes or some sweetened juice will usually correct the problem quickly until you can get to a health-care facility or contact your doctor. If the blood sugar goes so low that you become unconscious, you would be in a life-threatening situation, and it is essential that you be taken to a health-care facility where you can be given the necessary intravenous glucose to replace your blood sugar and start whatever other treatment you may need.

12 Emergency and Hospital Treatment of Asthma

I F YOUR asthma has gone increasingly out of control and continues to get worse in spite of following the instructions in *Chapter 11*, you will need treatment in a hospital casualty department. If the asthma attack is severe enough, you may need to be admitted to an intensive care unit until the problem has been brought under control.

In a severe attack, the airways are greatly narrowed by swelling, bronchoconstriction, and mucous plugging. It is like having to breathe through a drinking straw, and your diaphragm and chest wall muscles become increasingly exhausted. Thus, the ability to adequately ventilate the air sacs in the lungs falls. The result is that enough oxygen cannot get into the blood and carbon dioxide cannot be effectively removed. Unless the situation can be relieved quickly by following the detailed instructions in *Chapter 11* or by the doctors at the hospital, it may be necessary to help your breathing with a machine called a *ventilator*. If the initial treatment described in *Chapter 11* is successful in relieving the obstruction in the air passages, as it usually is, this should not be necessary.

SIGNS OF A VERY SEVERE AND LIFE-THREATENING ATTACK

Your asthma needs immediate attention if there is:

1. Severe shortness of breath even when sitting down or walking slowly that does not respond well to bronchodilator puffs, even after these have been administered repeatedly to the point of trembling or heart palpitations as detailed in *Chapter 11*.

2. Difficulty speaking because of breathlessness.

3. Difficulty sleeping, with repeated awakening at night and little relief from the bronchodilator inhalers.

4. Deterioration in peak flow readings by 30 to 50 percent (if you are monitoring these).

5. Increasing fear that you will not get enough breath.

6. Cold clamminess and weakness.

7. A bluish appearance to the tongue, lips, and fingertips.

8. Increasing exhaustion.

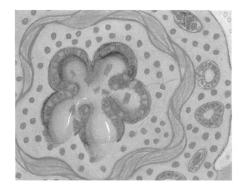

Note: It is impossible to tell the severity of an asthma attack by the amount of wheezing, because during a severe attack, the airways become so blocked that little or no sound is produced.

GETTING TO THE HOSPITAL

As part of your action plan, you should have worked out with your doctor exactly what to do up to now to try and avert deterioration of your asthma (see *Chapter 11*). Just as important is to develop an action plan for what to do if the asthma continues to deteriorate in spite of following these instructions.

At this point, you should go as quickly as possible to the nearest medical assistance — ideally a hospital casualty department, where the problem can be dealt with quickly, efficiently, and expertly. If your breathlessness is not yet severe, you can be driven to the hospital (you certainly should not drive yourself if you can possibly avoid it) by family car or taxi. If the asthma is more severe and seems to be deteriorating rapidly, you should call an ambulance. However, if an ambulance cannot pick you up quickly, you should get to the hospital by any means at your disposal as quickly as you can.

THE HOSPITAL CASUALTY DEPARTMENT

On arrival, if you are not extremely ill, you will talk briefly to a receptionist, who will record vital information. You will then be seen immediately by a nurse and/or doctor. If you are extremely ill on arrival, these formalities will be bypassed in order to start treatment at once. On arrival, show your medical summary card to the doctor or nurse, even without being asked for it (they may not know that you have one with you). This card provides vital information that will help the doctors to treat you and to avoid things that may make matters worse or cause side effects.

CASUALTY DEPARTMENT TREATMENT

After taking a brief history of the present attack and your previous experience with asthma (provided that you are well enough to give it), the doctor will do a quick but thorough physical examination, while starting treatment as follows:

1. Oxygen will be administered, usually by mask. The blood oxygen level will often be monitored by means of a device that fits on your finger or earlobe called an *oximeter*.

2. If possible, a breathing test such as the peak flow will be done at about the time treatment is started. The test will be repeated to see whether the treatment is working and to help your doctor decide whether you need to be admitted to the hospital or can be sent home later.

3. An arterial blood sample is often taken to tell how well oxygen is getting into your blood and to see whether your airways are so obstructed that you cannot get enough air into the air sacs to get rid of carbon dioxide. This is a good indication of how exhausted you have become and will help the doctor decide whether you need to be put on a breathing machine to give you a rest if, after providing treatment, there has not been the expected improvement.

4. Although you have probably taken numerous puffs from your inhaler before reaching the hospital, much of this has probably been wasted. Thus you will usually be given a large dose of bronchodilator aerosol from a nebulizer with a mask or alternatively you may be given several more bronchodilator puffs with a metered dose inhaler using a valved spacer device. This additional aerosol will only be given if you are not already trembling from

having given yourself many puffs and if irregularities of the heartbeat are not present (the doctors will be monitorying your heartbeat with an electrocardiograph while the treatment is going on). This should give you rapid partial relief of the breathlessness.

5. At the same time, you will receive intravenous fluid containing large doses of cortisone medication to reduce the inflammation. Alternatively you may be given a large dose of prednisolone tablets to swallow (usually 12). This is the most important part of the treatment after the initial bronchodilator puffs have opened your airways to some extent. It takes approximately 3 hours before this anti-inflammatory part of the treatment begins to have an effect.

   In the past, intravenous aminophylline was usually added, but this drug is now going out of favour because the aerosol inhalations usually provide the much-needed immediate relief and do so more quickly and effectively without the frequent side effects caused by aminophylline.

The aerosol bronchodilator may be provided by the same inhaler that you use at home, to which is usually added one of the valved spacer devices such as the Nebuhaler® or Volumatic®. This makes sure that you get some of the medication with each breath, even if you are panting quickly. Sometimes the bronchodilator inhaler provides relief so quickly that it is not necessary to give you the steroid treatment intravenously. Instead, you might be started on prednisolone tablets in large doses and observed for a suitable period to make sure that the asthma attack is getting better and will not return.

You will then often be sent home with instructions from your doctor to gradually taper the prednisolone tablets and resume the maintenance inhaled-steroid or other preventer treatment that kept you well before deterioration occurred. You should arrange to see your own doctor within a few days to make sure that you are improving steadily. If the previous maintenance treatment was not sufficient to keep your asthma under control because asthma attacks were occurring on a fairly regular basis, your whole treatment programme should be re-examined and the medication adjusted to bring you under better control, as outlined in *Chapter 11*.

ADMISSION TO HOSPITAL

If, in spite of the measures outlined above, you continue to deteriorate or fail to improve and particularly if:

1. You were admitted to the hospital within the last few days or weeks with a similarly severe asthma attack;
2. You have been taking steroid tablets at home recently;
3. You failed to show a considerable improvement in peak flow in response to large bronchodilator aerosol doses in the emergency department, or
4. You are afraid to be sent home,

your doctor will almost always admit you to hospital for further treatment and close observation.

The best place for you under these circumstances would be an intensive care unit, where you could be closely checked until the asthma is greatly improved.

If you continue to get worse in spite of the treatment outlined above, your breathing will need to be assisted by a mechanical ventilator. This is done by gently inserting a flexible plastic tube through your mouth and vocal cords into the windpipe, thus providing the airflow and oxygen that is lacking. The ventilator will give you a much needed

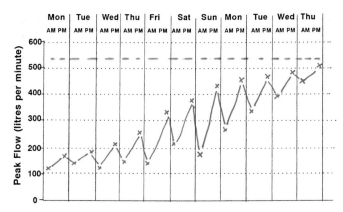

Peak flow chart showing recovery from an attack of asthma in hospital. Peak flow shows increased variability during recovery, reaching near normal values over several days.

rest, allow the exhausted diaphragm and chest wall muscles to recover their strength, and "buy time" for the anti-inflammatory steroid medications to begin to work. If at any stage in the treatment there is evidence of bacterial or other infection as well, appropriate antibiotics will be provided.

RECOVERING FROM SEVERE ATTACKS

If your asthma has been under control, episodes like the one described above should be extremely rare. However, such an attack may occur if a severe viral cold with bronchitis preceded deterioration of the asthma or if you were exposed to a large amount of the substance to which you are allergic. It is a rule of thumb that, even with vigorous treatment, it takes almost as long to return to normal after a bad asthma attack as it took for the attack to develop.

In any case, after you have greatly improved and before leaving the hospital, you should review with your doctor why and how the deterioration occurred so that similar episodes can be avoided in future. The main reason that asthma becomes severe is failure to recognize that you are getting into increasing difficulty. This results in failure to start treatment with increased steroids soon enough and in large enough doses. Having severe and life-threatening asthma attacks usually indicates failure to take the prescribed medication regularly or failure to take an adequate dose (e.g., forgetting to take the preventer medication in full doses) as prescribed. Nevertheless, deterioration to the point of hospitalization can almost always be averted if you start large doses of prednisolone as soon as you begin to notice deterioration.

Before leaving the hospital, make sure that you fully understand which medications you should be taking at home and how they should be taken so that the same problem does not occur again. Also make sure that you have adequate supplies of medications on hand at all times to deal with any situation, even when you are away from home on business or on holiday.

13 Aerosol Inhalers, Metered Dose Inhaler Spacer (Add-On) Devices, Nebulizers, and Oxygen Therapy

IT SHOULD be obvious to you by now (see *Chapters 10 and 11*) that the best way to treat asthma is to take anti-inflammatory (preventer) medications **regularly** and bronchodilator (reliever) medications **as required**, by inhaling medication aerosols. The best, most versatile, and cheapest way to take the inhalations is from a metered dose inhaler (MDI), which uses a tiny pressurised canister to create the aerosol spray, rather than from an expensive and cumbersome nebulizing machine. Some MDIs, called metered dose powder inhalers (MDPIs) provide powder aerosols on forced inhalation.

For the treatment to be effective you must use the MDI properly, or the medication will not get to your lungs. The proper use of an MDI involves five easy steps. You should review how you use the inhaler with your doctor and pharmacist to make sure that you are doing it properly. Children under the age of about four, the elderly, and those handicapped by strokes, rheumatoid arthritis, and other joint or muscle diseases, as well as asthmatics having a severe attack, may have difficulty using these devices properly, so a parent or close relative should make sure that the devices are being used properly.

HOW TO USE A METERED DOSE INHALER (MDI)

The steps are as follows:
1. Remove the cap from the plastic mouthpiece and shake the inhaler three or four times vigorously.
2. Breathe out in a relaxed way as though completing a sigh (there is no need to exhale forcibly or fully).
3. Hold the inhaler firmly, with the mouthpiece about two finger widths (4 cm) in front of your widely opened mouth. Direct the spray nozzle straight towards the back of the throat. (Perform these steps in front of a mirror until you are good at it!)
4. Breathe in slowly and completely, taking about 5 seconds to do so (like the beginning of a sigh). Just **after** beginning to breathe in, press the metal canister down firmly once to release the spray, which will then be taken into your lungs. Each push on the canister releases a precise dose. The canister should only be pushed **once** for each breath in.
5. After inhaling fully, hold your breath for up to 10 seconds, and then breathe out.
6. Take additional puffs one at a time, waiting about 60 seconds between each one, until you have taken the total number prescribed by your doctor.

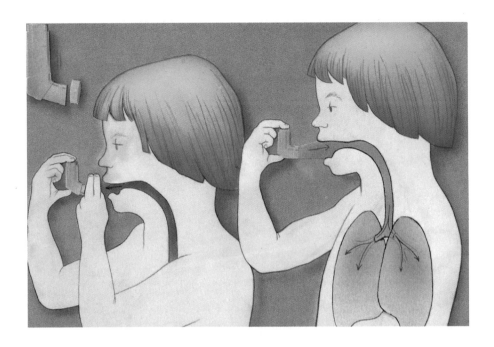

This technique is very important to follow in order to get the full dose of medication into your lungs.

ALTERNATIVE METHOD OF INHALING FROM A METERED DOSE INHALER

Some doctors and the labels packed with the inhalers suggest that the inhaler mouthpiece be put inside your mouth with your lips closed. This technique should only be used if you cannot use the open mouth method successfully, because you get much less of the medicine into your lungs.

NOTE: Perform these steps in front of a mirror to practice the correct technique. If the spray comes out of your mouth or nose like smoke, you are not inhaling correctly. Review the steps above and try again. If you are still having problems, see your doctor or pharmacist.

If in spite of good instruction and repeated attempts to use the inhaler properly, you are still having difficulty, ask your doctor whether you might benefit from one of the valved MDI accessory (add-on) holding chamber devices or a powder inhaler.

AUTOHALER

This device, developed by the Riker Company, has recently become available. Its main advantage is that it provides aerosol from a pressurised metered dose inhaler canister on demand as soon as you begin to breathe in. Thus, the need to coordinate aerosol discharge and inhalation is avoided. This device is almost foolproof, and because only a very gentle inhalation is required to trigger it, children over about age 3 or elderly people can easily use this inhaler to get their aerosol medication reliably. The disadvantage of this device is that, like all metered dose inhalers, about 90 percent of the drug is deposited at the back of the throat, with the potential for both local side effects and, because this medication may be absorbed into the body, widespread (but minor) side effects as well.

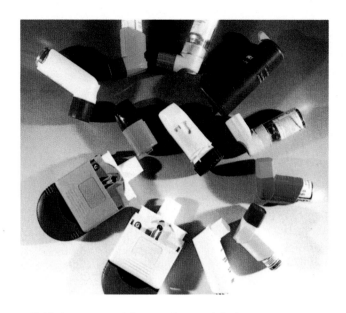

Inhalers are available in a range of shapes, sizes and designs.

By using this device together with a metered dose inhaler spacer device (see below), a fully automatic aerosol delivery system results that provides almost ideal targeting of the medication to the lungs, thus reducing side effects to an absolute minimum while providing the best possible and most reliable treatment of asthma.

METERED DOSE INHALER
SPACER (ADD-ON) DEVICES

Metered dose inhalers are the most versatile way of giving asthma medications, but some people are unable to coordinate discharge of the aerosol and breathing the aerosol into their lungs. Spacer devices have been developed to help assure aerosol delivery to the air passages. These devices (including Volumatic® or Nebuhaler®) have additional benefits as well (see Table 13–1, Benefits of Metered Dose Inhaler Spacer Devices). Besides helping to assure that the aerosol medicine gets to your lungs, add-on devices slightly increase the amount and improve the distribution of the inhaled medicine in your lungs. They also greatly reduce the amount of the spray that coats your mouth and throat, that part of the medication (75 percent) that never reaches your lungs but can be absorbed into your body. This allows a larger proportion of the medication to reach your air passages, increases the benefits of the medicine, and greatly reduces side effects, especially effects on the rest of your body from inhaled steroids when relatively large daily doses (over 1.5 mg of beclomethasone or equivalent) are used.

Spacer devices also reduce irritation of the tongue and throat and a fungus infection of the mouth, throat, and vocal cords (thrush) that sometimes results from inhaling steroids. Additional advantages are decreased gagging and cough and reduced taste of the inhaled medicine. Because some patients feel and taste very little of the spray in the back of their throat when the accessory devices are used, they incorrectly think that they are not getting the medication. However, if an accessory device is used correctly, you get the same or a little more medication than with a properly used ordinary inhaler.

POWDER INHALERS

Metered dose powder inhalers (MDPIs) (Rotahaler®, Diskhaler®, Spinhaler®, Turbohaler®) provide powder aerosol particles of the medication and have the advantage that the medicine is only released and inhaled when you breathe in. A potential problem with the powder inhaler devices is that during a bad attack, if you cannot inhale forcefully, you may get very little of the medication down into your lungs. Another problem is that powder inhalers do not reduce the side effects of the metered dose inhalers the way the addition of aerosol holding chambers to MDIs do. This is because 80–90 percent of the medicine still ends up at the back of your throat and around your vocal cords and much of it is absorbed, contributing unnecessarily to side effects if large doses of bronchodilators or inhaled steroids are used. In order to cut down side effects when steroid MDPIs are used, it is important to rinse the mouth with water immediately after use and spit out the fluid. This prevents any of the steroid in the mouth from being swallowed. MDPIs are not useful in children under 3 or 4 years who may not be able to suck hard enough to create the powder aerosol. If you blow into them before inhaling, all of the medicine will be lost. The new dry powder inhalers (Turbohaler®, Diskhaler®) which provide multiple doses are easier and more convenient to use. Many patients prefer these to MDIs. They do not cause the cough or throat irritation sometimes seen with MDI inhalers (due to the propellants).

NEBULIZERS

Aerosols have been used to treat lung disease for nearly a hundred years. Aerosols have been produced in a number of different ways. An example is the steam kettle, which is still used to humidify an infant's room during episodes of bronchitis or croup. About 50 years ago, a common treatment for asthma was aerosolized adrenaline. The aerosol was generated by air pressure using a squeeze bulb that the patient compressed vigorously to create the aerosol, which could then be inhaled from a glass tube.

Since then, nebulizers have become increasingly sophisticated. It is now possible to obtain a variety of these devices that make use of an electric air compressor to provide the force needed to aerosolize the drug solution within the nebulizer. Another common aerosol generating device is the ultrasonic nebulizer, which uses an electric current to stimulate a small crystal to vibrate at a high speed. This breaks the liquid solution up into small particles that are then inhaled as drug aerosol.

The advantage of nebulizers is that the drug is provided through a mask or mouthpiece while the patient is breathing normally. No particular skill is required. Until recently, this was the only way of giving aerosol to children under the age of 3 or 4, to frail, elderly or unconscious people and to patients on ventilator machines. Nebulizers remain the only way of providing certain drugs by aerosol (for example, antibiotics) that are not yet available as pressurized metered dose inhalers or powders. A main disadvantage is the expense of giving therapy in this way, because these delivery systems may cost a great deal of money, and the drug solutions are also much more expensive than puffs from a metered dose inhaler or inhalations from pow-

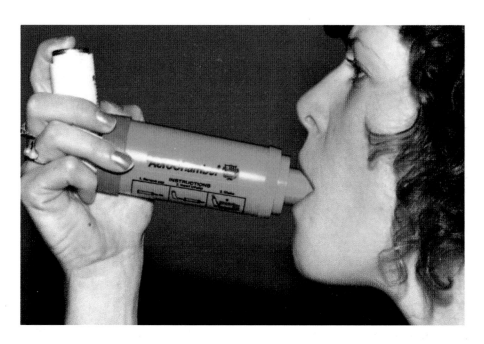

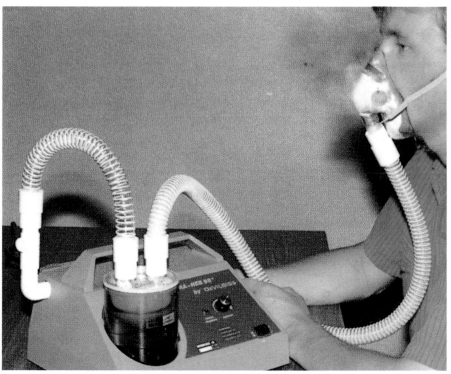

Metered-dose inhaler with add-on device (top) and a nebulizer (bottom).

der inhalers. The devices are also rather cumbersome and must be plugged into an electrical outlet (although recently, battery-operated units have been developed). Nebulizers are only about a third as efficient as metered dose inhalers, and very much larger doses of drugs are required to get an equivalent effect as compared to metered dose inhalers. Furthermore, not all drugs that are available as metered dose inhalers are yet available for use with nebulizers.

NEBULIZERS ARE NO BETTER THAN METERED DOSE INHALERS

Because, until fairly recently, nebulizers were the devices most commonly used in hospital emergency departments and on the wards, patients thought that aerosol therapy with nebulizers was somehow superior to treatments with metered dose inhalers. The only reason that this was so is that **much larger doses** of the bronchodilator medications were provided in nebulizers for treating severe episodes of asthma in the emergency department while patients were in hospital, and so the response to treatment was better. **The improvement was a result of the larger dose and not the delivery system**.

A number of recent scientific studies have shown that the metered dose inhaler together with a spacer device is actually superior to nebulizers because of the ability of the MDI to provide treatment more rapidly and at much lower cost than nebulizer treatments. Of course, at the time of a severe asthma attack, more puffs than usual will be needed (see *Chapter 11*). Another advantage of the MDI and spacer device is that it can be easily carried with you, and so effective treatment, even for severe asthma, is available to you or your child (using the Nebuhaler® with mask) wherever you may be.

Because the metered dose inhaler together with an accessory device is an effective and low-cost aerosol delivery system that has been shown in many studies to be as good or better than nebulizers, hospitals have discontinued the use of nebulizers for treating children and adults and many more are likely to switch over in the future. Doing this results in substantial savings annually to an average city hospital, a great boon at a time of ever tighter budgets!

About 20 years ago, the use of positive pressure machines for "pushing" aerosols into the lungs was popular, but these systems are hardly used any more, except in patients who require assisted ventilation because they cannot breathe adequately themselves. Research has shown that these systems are even less efficient than nebulizers and are therefore much less useful than MDIs and spacer devices. Indeed, a new device called the AeroVent® now allows the use of metered dose inhalers even with ventilator machines in hospital intensive care units and for the occasional patients who use ventilators to assist their breathing at home.

OXYGEN TREATMENT IN ASTHMA: WHEN, WHY, AND HOW

In contrast to patients with chronic bronchitis and emphysema, who may require oxygen at night, during exercise, or between 15 and 24 hours a day when the disease is severe, most patients with well-controlled asthma do not require oxygen except during life-threatening attacks. However, with time, patients with poorly controlled asthma may develop marked and relatively permanent narrowing of their airways, particularly if they have also been smokers for many years. Oxygen may then be necessary.

Oxygen therapy should only be prescribed by your doctor, who will often

HOW MUCH MEDICATION IS LEFT?

FULL	HALF	EMPTY
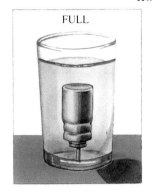	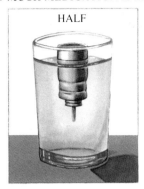	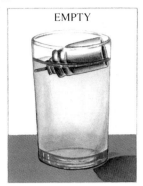

A simple test to check your bronchodilator supply.

seek the advice of a lung specialist. Oxygen therapy is used to provide enough additional oxygen to supply the needs of your body's cells. There is no point taking extra oxygen if the blood is already adequately supplied by the air around you. Your doctor can arrange tests to find out whether extra oxygen is needed. These tests are often used to find out whether adequate oxygen gets to the blood on exercise and at night. The oxygen levels in your blood may be adequate when you are sitting quietly, but this does not guarantee that the levels will be adequate when you are asleep or are exercising even moderately (or flying in an airplane).

The amount of oxygen needed when levels in your blood are too low is the amount of oxygen that will restore near normal levels in your blood (over 94 percent oxygen saturation), provided that you are not chronically retaining the waste gas carbon dioxide in your system. If you do chronically retain carbon dioxide, then oxygen administration must be carried out very carefully by means of a controlled oxygen mask and only under the supervision of a doctor who fully understands how to treat this sort of problem.

Oxygen can be provided at home by oxygen cylinders which, in recent years, have usually been replaced by far more convenient oxygen concentrators. Oxygen concentrators are small electrical machines that look and behave almost like a small refrigerator. They extract oxygen from the air to provide it to you at the concentrations you require.

Portable oxygen systems are now

TABLE 13–1 BENEFITS OF METERED DOSE INHALER SPACER DEVICES

1. Assure aerosol delivery to airways in infants, children, and adults.
2. Reduce side effects in the mouth and throat (hoarseness, and fungus infection).
3. Reduce total body steroid dose thus allowing larger doses to the airways safely.
4. Reduce side effects throughout the body.
5. Replace expensive and cumbersome nebulizers for most adults and children.

readily available. They consist of a small tank weighing about 12 pounds that you can carry over your shoulder. The tank provides portable oxygen for about 2 to 4 hours and can be refilled from a liquid oxygen supply that you keep in a large cylinder at home.

Oxygen is usually taken by mask or, more conveniently, by nasal prongs. Lately oxygen delivery has been made less obvious for some patients by inserting a small plastic tube through the windpipe near the root of the neck and burying it under the skin of the chest wall so that it can be connected to an oxygen supply near the belt line.

Fortunately, people with asthma rarely require oxygen as long as the condition is kept under good control, as outlined in *Chapter 11*.

It goes without saying and is well worth repeating here that adding cigarette smoke (even second hand smoke) to asthma is adding serious insult to airway injury. This includes parents smoking in the vicinity of their asthmatic children!

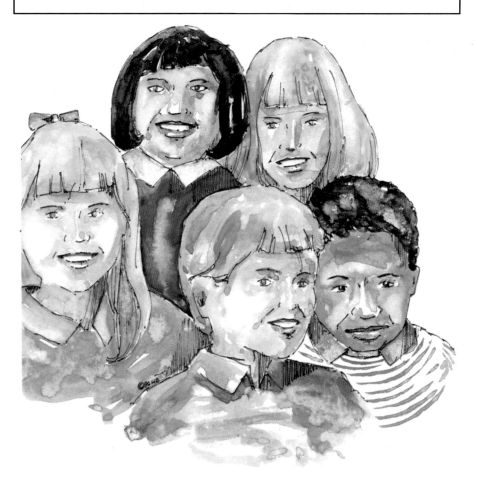

HOW COMMON?

Asthma is the most common chronic disease in childhood, affecting at least 10 percent of all children. It seems to be more common in boys than girls (but this is not the case in adults). Asthma usually improves during adolescence, but about half of such children develop asthma again as adults—although there is often a period in the late teens and twenties when asthma goes away completely.

SPECIAL FEATURES OF CHILDHOOD ASTHMA

Although asthma in children is, in many ways, similar to asthma in adults, there are certain special features. Asthma in infants and children is often diagnosed as "wheezy bronchitis" when wheezing appears to come on after what seem to be recurring chest infections. It is often treated repeatedly and incorrectly with antibiotics. Furthermore, there was, in the

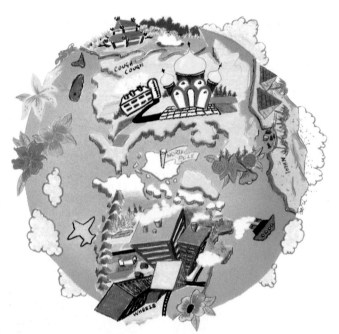

past, a reluctance to use the term "asthma" because parents were frightened by the thought that their child might have a serious and chronic illness. If a child has several episodes of "wheezy bronchitis" one after the other, this is almost always asthma.

Coughing may be the most obvious symptom of asthma in children. A dry or mucousy cough at night is common and is often not diagnosed as asthma because the child may not complain of shortness of breath and may not wheeze. Coughing and wheezing after exercise are also common in asthmatic children — mainly because children run about more than adults. Crying can also set off wheezing, as can laughter.

Asthma in children is usually, but not necessarily, allergic in nature. Children often develop wheezing after exposure to allergic triggers such as animals. Some children only get asthma symptoms after contact with horses, cats, or dogs, although symptoms that are specific to only one animal are unusual. Cats are a common problem and feather-filled

comforters (duvets, eiderdowns) may require you and your doctor to be Sherlock Holmes and Dr Watson to sleuth out the cause of your child's night-time asthma attacks. Seasonal asthma is common in children, and so is exercise-induced asthma, which may cause major psychological problems because, unable to participate in sports and many other activities, poorly controlled asthmatic children may become lonely and withdrawn.

Children with asthma often have other allergic problems, called hay fever (in the pollen season) or runny nose (rhinitis) at any time of year. Rhinitis, especially when it comes and goes throughout the year, may be diagnosed as frequent "colds." The skin of asthmatic children may be affected by eczema, particularly the areas in front of the elbows and wrists, and behind the knees.

Not surprisingly, many parents think that their child is particularly susceptible to "colds" that "seem to go to the chest." Such frequently recurring episodes, which seem to come one after the other, are almost always caused by asthma and rhinitis. These episodes respond well to asthma treatment but antibiotics and cough medicines are not usually very effective.

Conjunctivitis (itchy eyes) may also be a major problem for your child; indeed, the first clue to cat or dog allergy may be swollen red eyes when your child plays with the pet and then touches their eyes.

GROWING OUT OF ASTHMA

Studies that have followed asthmatic children as they develop all suggest that many children improve. Between 60–80% of children with asthma are free of symptoms at adolescence. Children with mild asthma that does not need regular treatment nearly all become symptom-free, whereas children with troublesome asthma requiring regular treatment and frequent hospital admissions often have persistent asthma. In adult life, those who have had asthma in childhood may get symptoms back again after a symptom-free period of several years. As many as half of the people who have asthma during childhood will develop asthma at some time during adulthood.

TREATING CHILDHOOD ASTHMA

The principles of treating childhood asthma are the same as for asthma in adults.

Most important of all is avoidance of identified (or suspected) allergic factors if possible. Parents should eliminate cigarette (or other) smoking in the house. Children with allergic asthma should not have close contact with pets, such as cats, to which they may be allergic. Some children will also benefit from annual influenza vaccine. If all else fails, controlling asthma, rhinitis, and conjunctivitis with medication is essential for the future health and emotional well-being of your child.

A combination of bronchodilators and anti-inflammatory drugs is used. For mild and infrequent asthma, such as occasional wheezing after exercise, an inhaled beta-agonist bronchodilator such as salbutamol (Ventolin), preferably taken before the exercise, is all that is usually needed.

Which bronchodilator? The choice is the same as for adults: beta-agonist inhalers are best. Theophylline is a

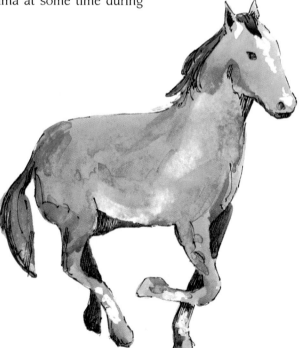

weak bronchodilator (reliever) and has problems with side effects. In children, anticholinergics (like Atrovent) only rarely work.

Side effects from theophylline may be troublesome in children, as in adults, but recently learning and behavioural difficulties have been found in children taking even the correct doses. Theophylline should nowadays only be considered third line therapy and is rarely needed if the almost side effect-free anti-inflammatory 'preventers' and beta-agonist inhalers (relievers) are used in effective doses.

Which anti-inflammatory drug? Of the anti-inflammatory treatments, cromoglycate, which is inhaled, is the drug of first choice if the asthma is moderate in severity. It has no side effects and it is effective in many children, particularly if there is a strong allergic background. If taken 15 minutes before exercise it is also effective in preventing exercise-induced asthma if the bronchodilators alone have not done the trick. Unfortunately, cromoglycate needs to be taken four times a day to give the best protection against asthma and this can prove to be a problem with children at school. It is more expensive and less effective than the more powerful inhaled steroids.

Inhaled steroids work as well in children as in adults and, in low doses, do not cause side effects because not enough of the drug is absorbed into the body to cause problems. Although steroid tablets are known to cause stunting of growth in children, this has not been shown with the low doses from steroid inhalers (under 500 μg daily) — in fact, children tend to increase their growth, since severe asthma that is not well controlled can delay growth. By using MDIs plus a spacer device, a much larger asthma controlling dose can be used safely because absorption into the blood-stream from the mouth and stomach is greatly reduced by the spacer. So inhaled steroids, under careful supervision of a doctor, work well in children and give good control of asthma. Because inhaled steroids usually need to be given only twice a day, it is much easier for parents to supervise the treatment. Metered dose inhaler spacers, such as the Nebuhaler® or Volumatic®, should always be used with inhaled steroids, because these decrease side effects by reducing the local dose to the throat and voice box and the total body dose to about a quarter of what it would be otherwise.

Steroid tablets are used long term only in the most severe cases of asthma. As in adults, the lowest dose needed to control symptoms should be given on alternate days, if possible, together with other medications as needed to limit the dose of tablets to an absolute minimum. Any child taking high doses of inhaled steroid (over 500 μg/day) or who needs steroid tablet treatment should be under the care of a specialist so that asthma control, growth and any side effects can be carefully monitored.

INHALERS OR TABLETS?

The conventional inhaler may be difficult for small children (under the age of 5) to use correctly because of the need to coordinate release of the spray to breathing in. Dry powder inhalers (e.g. Turbohalers or Rotahalers) are easier for children over 4 or 5 years old to use. However, powder inhalers may not work during severe attacks because high flows are needed to release the powder. Both bronchodilators (e.g., Ventolin and Bricanyl) and anti-inflammatory drugs (e.g., Intal, Becotide, Pulmicort) can be given in this way, and the new powder devices are easy to use. Multidose dry powder inhalers (MDPIs), particularly the Turbohaler®, are easy for children to use, and a good way to give inhaled steroids to children. A valved accessory device for use with MDIs (see *Chapter 13*) may be particularly useful, since the older child or parent can activate the inhaler into the aerosol holding chamber, and then the child can breathe in through the one-way valve. New aerosol inhalation systems with a mask allow inhalers to be used in infants and children under 3 years old.

Powder inhalers cannot be used with spacer devices, otherwise most of the medication would be deposited in the throat increasing the likelihood of side effects.

Nebulizers may be useful in children who have severe attacks if multiple puffs from the bronchodilator inhaler delivered by a spacer with a mask are not fully effective. In this way parents are able to deal with the attack at home, which is much better for the child (and the parents) psychologically.* Children with asthma severe enough to require nebulizers should always be under the care of a specialist so that the correct preventative treatment can be worked out. The metered dose inhaler spacers with a valve can usually replace nebulizers, and provide similarly effective therapy with much greater convenience and at much lower cost.

Children are often embarrassed by having to use an inhaler device, especially at school. This often prevents them from taking the treatment they need. At some schools the treatment has to be given by a teacher, and this even further inhibits the child from taking regular treatment. That is why in-

* Following such an attack, additional treatment with prednisolone tablets is usually needed, so your doctor should be contacted as soon as possible. If the episode recurs or persists, you should take your child to the closest healthcare facility **without delay**. Having attacks indicates that the asthma is out of control (see *Chapter 11*). This situation **must be corrected** at once since it could lead to life-threatening asthma.

haled steroids, given twice a day at home before and after school are usually the best way of controlling asthma in children. In addition, children should also carry a bronchodilator MDI with them for self care of asthma attacks, if they are old enough to do so reliably. If not, an appropriate care giver at kindergarten or day-care should be instructed in the proper use of MDIs and necessary accessory devices.

TAKING MEDICINES BY MOUTH

Children don't like taking tablets, but some bronchodilators can be given in the form of syrups. Previously, these syrups contained sugar and artificial colours, but now an artificial sweetener has been substituted. For some theophylline preparations, a "sprinkle" has been developed that is sprinkled onto food and seems to give the right dose. As a general rule aerosols are much more effective than swallowed medicines and rarely cause side effects. **Whenever possible aerosols should be used to treat asthma in infants and children.**

ASTHMA IN BABIES

Asthma in babies is often difficult to diagnose and treat. It may be difficult to make the diagnosis because measurements are not easy to make. In the past, treatment was a problem because babies were unable to use inhalers. However, nebulizers can now be used to deliver most drugs. Beta-agonist inhalers are almost as effective as in older children or adults, and anticholinergics may be useful in some babies. Inhaled steroids, which can be given by nebulizer, are becoming available and initial reports suggest that they will be useful in this age group. Recently, valved aerosol spacer chambers with a mask (e.g., Nebuhaler® with mask) have been developed that

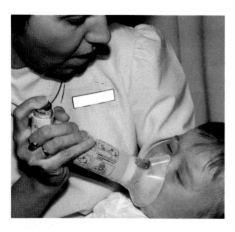

A special bronchodilator for baby.

can be attached to all inhalers and allow virtually any of these spray medications to be given to infants and children under 3 years of age (see *Chapter 13*).

How Should Parents Cope with Asthmatic Children?

Parents are naturally worried when they learn that their child suffers from asthma. This is mainly because people often have the wrong impression of the condition. Asthma is not a "nervous" or neurotic disease, and having asthma does not mean that a child has psychological problems. Of course, stress and worry can trigger asthma attacks if the condition is poorly controlled (as discussed in *Chapter 8*), but this is only one of many triggers. Parents often feel guilty and frightened that their child has asthma, and this may create a stressful situation at home that may make the asthma worse. Parents should not have a sense of guilt about their child's asthma; the condition is never due to something the parents have or haven't done but is an illness, like any other, that almost always responds well to proper treatment.

How should you cope with asthma in your child? The simplest answer is that you should treat your son or daughter as a **normal** child. With proper treatment, asthma can almost always be controlled so that your child can do almost everything just like his/her age mates. This means taking part in all sports activities (sometimes using the bronchodilator inhaler before exercise). One exception is scuba diving which is potentially dangerous, even for well-controlled asthmatics.

Family pets may be a problem if a child is allergic to them, and it may be advisable not to introduce new pets into the home (apart from fish!). It is often difficult to get rid of a loved family pet, and this might cause so much distress that the asthma actually gets worse. If the pet stays, direct **contact** with the animal must be avoided – and pets must **never** sleep in the same bedroom as the child with asthma or near the heating system air intake during the winter.

You should supervise the treatment to make sure your child is using the inhalers properly and at the right time. Children usually hate taking any sort of treatment, so you must be persistent and encouraging. Some children find that keeping a chart is helpful, as it gives them a feeling of helping in the control of their condition. Many children are carefree rather than careless about dealing with their asthma. A charming and intelligent twelve-year-old girl that we cared for, whose asthma was poorly controlled because she often forgot to take her medication, attached her steroid inhaler to the handle of her toothbrush with a rubber band to remind her to take her puffs twice a day. Her asthma is now exceptionally well controlled, and she leads a normal, active life.

COPING AT SCHOOL

Most children with asthma can cope normally at school, and no special arrangements need to be made. In the past it was common for children with asthma to often be absent from school, but nowadays, with much better treatment available, this is rarely necessary. Children with asthma should be encouraged to participate in as many school sports as they wish. Sometimes sprinting is difficult but, if the bronchodilator inhaler is taken 10 minutes before exercise, there should not be any problems. The same applies to cross-country running, skiing, or hockey. Swimming is often the best tolerated exercise in children who have troublesome asthma.

Many children are embarrassed about having asthma and are reluctant to use their inhalers in class. It is particularly upsetting for a child to have to ask the teacher for the inhaler. It is much better if children can keep the inhaler with them (if they do so at home). The teacher should know that a child has asthma, particularly if troublesome attacks occur. Ideally, your doctor should write to the school explaining the condition and requesting that the child control inhaler use. A few children with **very severe** asthma may benefit from attending a special school and summer camp for asthmatic children, where special facilities are available. However, the need for such schools is now rare, since asthma is so much better controlled with preventer inhalers.

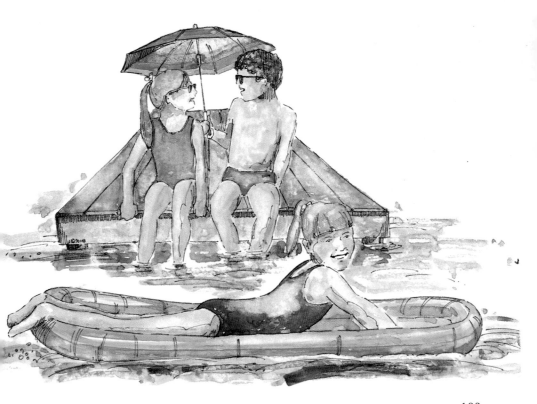

How should you cope with asthma in your child? The simplest answer is that you should treat your son or daughter as a **normal** child.

CASE STUDY

Mary was a 17-year-old girl with allergic asthma. Prior to coming to the chest clinic, she had missed 30 days of school in the previous year because of asthma, had given up football and other sports that she thoroughly enjoyed, had been forced to go to the hospital emergency department on six occasions in the previous 3 months for nebulizer treatments, and had been hospitalized for about 10 days. Her asthma was badly out of control. Not surprisingly, she had become withdrawn and depressed. She was on many different medications, including two types of bronchodilator (reliever) inhalers, a theophylline medication, and an anti-allergic (preventer) drug (cromoglycate), but in spite of all of this, she continued to have attacks.

At her first clinic assessment, Mary was found to be very sensitive to pollen and house dust on skin testing. She was given advice about avoiding the things to which she was allergic and was started on relatively large doses of inhaled steroids, which she was advised to take three times daily, preceded by an inhaled bronchodilator using metered dose inhalers and an accessory device. She kept a peak flow record, which in the first week showed an improvement in flow from around 300 L/min to about 450 L/min, which is her normal value. The marked swings (over 30% variation) in peak flow that had been present previously from morning to evening and from day to day disappeared, indicating that she was coming under much better control. She did not require any of the other medications that she had been taking prior to her first clinic visit.

With the onset of the grass pollen season, she began to play football more often and began having severe attacks once again, usually related to playing football, although she was reasonably well the rest of the time. When these attacks occurred, the young woman and her family became extremely upset and panicky, and when four puffs of the bronchodilator inhaler failed to give her relief, they rushed her to the hospital emergency department. There she was given a nebulizer containing the same bronchodilator medication (Ventolin). She gradually improved over the next hour annd was sent home without any additional medication.

Mary's mother phoned her doctor at the asthma clinic, very alarmed that her daughter was again having so much difficulty. Mary was advised to take a short course of prednisolone to bring the situation under better control and to increase the steroid inhaler dose to two puffs three times a day throughout the pollen season. She was advised to take four puffs of the bronchodilator medication **before exercise**, and if in spite of this she should have an attack of asthma, she was to use multiple bronchodilator puffs from her metered dose inhaler with a valved aerosol holding chamber (as detailed in *Chapters 11 and 13*), instead of rushing to the hospital emergency department. She was also advised to contact her own doctor immediately if this were necessary and to go to the emergency department if symptoms persisted.

Unfortunately, Mary did not follow the instructions to double the steroid inhaler dose to two puffs three times a day. She again got into severe difficulty while playing football at a park far from a hospital. By following the instructions in *Chapter 11*, she eventually took 18 puffs of the bronchodilator inhaler, over about 15 minutes, which completely reversed the asthma attack. Mild tremor was the only side effect.

When she was seen by the doctor the following day, she had herself started the prednisolone tablets as she was told to do if she had a severe episode, her peak flow readings which dropped to 200 L/ min during the attack, were again 370 L/min, and she was feeling almost normal. On reviewing what had happened with Mary and her parents, it seemed clear that she had got into difficulty because she did not follow the instructions in *Chapter 11* and on her wallet card, namely that when deterioration occurs and the peak flow drops, the steroid inhalations should be doubled. This should be continued for 1 week after symptoms disappear and the peak flow again returns to the previous level. After that, the number of daily puffs of steroid aerosol should be decreased to the previous maintenance dose under the doctor's close supervision.

During the pollen season, much more of the pollen allergen is inhaled, particularly on exercise, causing a more severe allergic reaction and more marked asthma. Mary was advised that she may find it necessary to continue the larger dose of the steroid inhaler throughout the pollen season, and she may well require four puffs rather than two of the bronchodilator medication before playing football. If doing this is not fully successful, then adding 2 to 4 puffs of cromoglycate before exercise to the bronchodilator (see *Chapters 10 and 11*) will usually prevent an attack of asthma.

This discussion with Mary and her parents obviously relieved much of their anxiety about asthma attacks, particularly since they were able to bring the problem under control themselves with the bronchodilator inhaler in a setting where no nebulizer was available. This also gave the opportunity to emphasize some important points about asthma treatment, namely that the dose of the preventer medications must be increased at the times that Mary is at increased risk of asthma attacks because of increased exposure to allergens (the same would be true if she were exposed to cats or horses, since she is allergic to both of these). Furthermore, Mary should use the bronchodilator inhaler and a cromoglycate inhaler about 15 minutes before exposure to these animals, not only to prevent the immediate airway constriction but also to block the so-called "late allergic reaction" that leads to prolonged inflammation (see *Chapter 5*). The doctor also explained the importance of the **dose** of medication and the need to take the larger protective dose of steroid inhalations **regularly** during the allergy season, which unfortunately Mary had not been doing. The doctor again went over with Mary that asthma is inflammation of the airways, and that in order to stay well and lead a normal life, it was necessary for her to meet the disease head on with effective treatment. Subsequently her asthma has remained well controlled for the most part. Flare-ups have been appropriately treated by Mary herself without the need for hospitalization.

Editorial Note: Teenagers can be the most difficult asthmatics to treat because they deny that they have a chronic problem and so "forget" to take their medication when they are feeling reasonably well. This denial is mixed with a great deal of anxiety and depression, which parents and doctors **must** understand in order to treat teenagers effectively. Mary and her parents were told that they could contact the clinic **at any time** for help should they have problems or questions. Such a "hot line" staffed by doctors should be available to asthmatics around the clock at every major treatment centre.

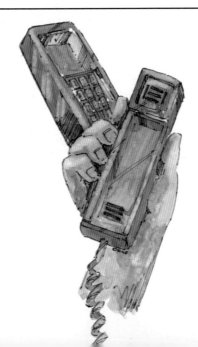

15 Noses, Ears, Eyes, and Asthma

I F YOU have asthma, it will be no surprise to you that this condition may be associated with problems outside the air passages of the lungs. The eyes, eyelids, and the nose are directly affected by the same allergic factors that injure the air passages of the lungs, because they are lined by similar tissues and are also directly exposed to the environment that contains the allergens. The sinuses and space within the middle ear are often injured by infection that results from inflammatory swelling of the tissues inside the nose and obstruction to the drainage of secretions from the sinuses and middle ear spaces. As with asthma, these problems may be caused by allergens (e.g., hay fever caused by ragweed) or to nonallergic factors, such as virus infections, that are still incompletely understood.

THE NOSE

The nose can be thought of as the gatekeeper of the lungs. Injury to the lining of the nose may be allergic or nonallergic, just as in the airways of the lungs. The resulting inflammation is called *rhinitis*. Typically there is swelling and excessive mucous secretion. If the problem is ongoing, additional long-term changes take place in the lining of the nose, leading to overgrowth of grape-like clusters of inflamed tissue called *nasal polyps*. These add to the obstruction of the nasal air passages and may contribute to plugging of the sinus openings. This prevents the sinuses from properly draining, resulting in infection — a condition called *sinusitis*. Because the middle ear space drains into the back of the throat through delicate narrow canals called the *eustachian tubes*, swelling of the tissues in the throat compresses' the tubes and causes clogging. This may lead to the recurring middle ear infections, called otitis media, that often occur in children.

Such problems may occur in the absence of asthma or may precede the onset of asthma by months or years. If these problems come and go often in children along with frequent episodes of cough or wheeziness, asthma and its consequences should be suspected.

If these problems begin in childhood, allergies are nearly always the cause and should be carefully investigated. The most important common allergens include cats, dogs, gerbils, hamsters, birds or bird feathers in duvets and pillows, and house dust containing the house dust mite. These mites flourish in humid and warm conditions, especially in bedding and carpets. All of these allergens are more likely to cause problems during the winter when the house is closed up, people tend to spend more of their time indoors, and the heating system blows the allergens about. In the spring, summer and autumn symptoms are much more likely to be pollen- or mould-related. Food allergy only rarely accounts for these problems.

If these diseases begin in adulthood, allergies are almost never the cause. It is thought that viruses somehow start the persistent inflammation in these cases.

Another form of rhinitis results from

irritation of the nerves in the lining of the nose, causing large amounts of thin, watery secretion. This is called *vasomotor rhinitis* and tends to occur in older people. This form of rhinitis is probably **not** associated with inflammation but occurs because of excessive responsiveness of the nerve endings in the nose, which leads to stimulation of the mucous glands and an outpouring of secretion.

CONTROLLING CONJUNCTIVITIS, RHINITIS, AND SINUSITIS

CONJUNCTIVITIS

Inflammation of the lining of the eyelids is known as *conjunctivitis*. This problem can be caused by bacterial infection, viruses, or allergens. It is very often caused by a reaction to allergens such as cats and is a common and annoying part of hay fever.

HOW TO RECOGNIZE CONJUNCTIVITIS

1. The eyes are red, swollen, and/or itchy.
2. The eyes contain pus (a thick yellow fluid consisting mainly of white blood cells associated with the inflammation).

HOW TO CONTROL ALLERGIC CONJUNCTIVITIS

1. Avoid the allergens if possible.
2. If the problem is mild to moderate, antihistamine drops (2 drops every 6 hours) or tablets should be used. (There are new varieties that do not make you drowsy). If the problem is more severe, cromoglycate drops (Opticrom, 2 drops every 4–6 hours) should be used to combat the inflammation. If the problem is very severe, prednisolone tablets may be needed for a few days to correct the situation, followed by the treatments outlined above to

keep the conjunctivitis under control.
3. If the conjunctivitis is associated with bacterial infection, an antibiotic will be needed.

RHINITIS

HOW TO RECOGNIZE RHINITIS

Rhinitis is inflammation of the lining of the nose that may be caused by the same things that cause conjunctivitis. The features of rhinitis include the following:
1. Sneezing
2. Itching
3. Swelling of the lining of the nose
4. Mucous plugging
5. Runniness
6. Postnasal drip causing bothersome and sleep-robbing cough.

Rhinitis often flares up at the same time as asthma. Since treating the asthma with aerosols has only a local effect in the air passages of the lungs, asthma treatment will have no beneficial effect on the nose.

HOW TO CONTROL RHINITIS

1. Avoid as much as possible the things that may be causing rhinitis, including allergens, irritants such as wood or metal dust, and people with viral illnesses such as colds or the 'flu'.
2. If allergic rhinitis (e.g., hay fever) is severe, bringing it under control may at first require a short course of prednisolone along with decongestants such as pseudoephedrine taken by mouth. If the nose is badly plugged and you cannot breathe through it, vasoconstrictor nose drops such as oxymetazoline (Otrivin) may be needed. Vasoconstrictor nose drops may cause rebound swelling after a short time and may injure the lining of the nose over the long term, so they

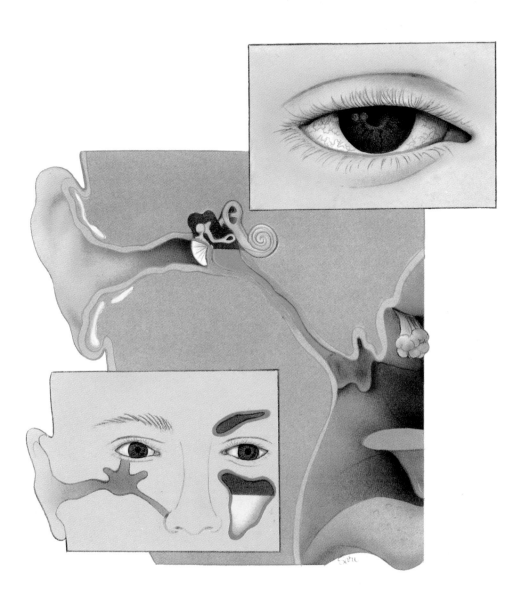

should only be used for a few days to clear the nasal passages and to assist drainage of the sinuses if these are clogged.

If the problem recurs often or is present most of the time then you will need long-term inhaled preventer medication such as nasal steroids (Beconase, Rhinocort and Flixonase), just as with asthma treatment. The usual dose is two puffs (50 μg per puff) into each nostril twice a day, although much larger doses are sometimes needed. An alternative treatment for mild rhinitis is cromoglycate (Rynacrom), inhaled 2 to 4 times a day into the nose. Cromoglycate is particularly useful for allergic rhinitis and is, at present, the only nasal medication available that will block the allergic reaction if taken about 15 minutes before exposure (for example, if you are going to visit a friend with a cat and you are allergic to cats). If your rhinitis is seasonal and you can easily identify approximately when it starts and stops, the best treatment consists in starting the preventer medicines (cromoglycate or inhaled steroids) when the allergy season begins and continuing on a regular daily basis until a week or two after the allergy season is over.

When steroids are sprayed into the nose, especially if large doses (over 400 μg daily) are needed, the lining of the air passages in the nose may become injured. Nose bleeds may result. Rarely the skin-like area inside the nose near the tip may develop erosions. The cartilage may then be badly injured. This may lead to a perforation between the two nasal passages. To try to avoid these problems the nasal spray should always be directed **away** from the nasal partition.

ALLERGY INJECTIONS

In contrast to asthma, which generally responds poorly to allergy injections (immunotherapy), the treatment of allergic rhinitis with injections has met with somewhat greater success, but mainly for treating hay fever. Desensitization with injections is bothersome because they often have to be taken over a period of 2 or 3 years. Furthermore, benefits are variable, with some people getting much more response than others, while other people do not seem to respond at all. Another problem associated with injection treatments are the local side effects, which consist mainly of swelling where the injections are given. Occasionally, severe generalized reactions (*anaphylaxis*) occur, which may cause serious illness or even death.

We rarely use injection treatment for these reasons and prefer to treat allergic rhinitis with the simple, effective, and usually safe treatments outlined above.

NASAL POLYPS

Nasal polyps are the result of severe longstanding inflammation of the lining of the nasal passages and consist of grape-like clusters of swollen lining tissue that fill the passages, more or less blocking them, and often obstructing the sinus drainage openings. This in turn may lead to infected sinuses (*sinusitis*), because the excessive secretions resulting from the inflammatory process become infected with bacteria, leading to collections of pus within the sinus cavities. These bacterial infections must be treated by encouraging drainage of the sinus fluid with decongestants and by the use of large doses of antibiotics, often for several weeks.

REMOVING NASAL POLYPS

Since well-established nasal polyps only sometimes respond completely, even to the most vigorous treatment with anti-inflammatory medicines, it is often necessary to remove the tissue surgically. Ear, nose and throat specialists usually perform these relatively minor operations. The result of the operation is an open nasal passage that allows you to breathe freely. However, the lining of the nose usually continues to become inflamed and swell after the polyps have been removed. If nothing is done to treat this recurring inflammation, polyps will usually form again within months or years and may have to be removed repeatedly. To prevent this from happening (or to at least slow down the process), steroid sprays should be used regularly in the nose. However, the dose to the nose is generally less than that required in the lungs to keep asthma under control.

The preventer medicines used to control symptoms in the nose may be given as puffs of inhaled steroids or cromoglycate from a metered dose inhaler, sprayed droplets from a pump-like device, or less commonly, as a powder that is blown into the nose with a squeeze bulb or sniffed in. Sometimes surgery of polyps can be avoided by using a short course of high dose prednisolone tablets to "shrink" the polyps, after which steroid sprays are used to try to keep the problem under control.

SINUSITIS

Sinusitis is inflammation of the lining of the hollow areas in the skull, called *sinuses*, which communicate with the inside of the nose through small openings. It is these small openings that are at the root of sinus problems. When the openings become swollen because of inflammation caused by allergies or other triggers, they narrow down or become completely clogged, so that the secretions in the sinuses cannot escape. Infection is usually the result.

HOW TO RECOGNIZE SINUSITIS

1. Plugged, congested nose that produces a thick yellow or green discharge, sometimes with blood in it when you blow your nose.
2. Dripping of the same secretions down the back of your throat, which irritates the vocal cords and causes cough and expectoration of phlegm similar to that coming out of your nose. The cough may be particularly severe at night.
3. Fever is common.
4. Pain in the face, which may be severe.
5. If neglected, sinusitis may lead to severe problems such as meningitis, which is infection of the membranes surrounding the brain tissue, an abscess of the brain tissue, or occasionally clotting of the veins in the head. These conditions are extremely serious and can lead to severe stroke-like disability or even death. Sinusitis should never be neglected, but prompt and vigorous treatment should be undertaken to relieve the congestion and eliminate the infection with antibiotics.

HOW TO CONTROL SINUSITIS

If recurring sinusitis cannot be prevented by vigorous long-term treatment of chronic rhinitis as outlined above, surgery may be needed, not only to remove nasal polyps, but also sometimes to enlarge the drainage opening from the sinuses. This allows the accumulated fluid to drain more freely. Sometimes the tonsils and/or adenoids, which may be so swollen that they block normal drainage openings, will need to be removed. An ear, nose and throat specialist will usually need to be consulted about these aspects of treatment.

Controlling sinusitis is also important because it is much harder to control asthma in people whose sinusitis is not under good control. Be sure to tell your doctor if you think you have sinusitis, so that it can be treated effectively.

MIDDLE EAR INFECTION (OTITIS MEDIA)

This condition commonly occurs in children with allergic rhinitis because the eustachian canals from the middle ear to the throat become plugged, and fluid accumulates in the space behind the ear drums. The resulting hearing impairment may result in poor performance in school. If the fluid becomes infected, fever, pain, and greater hearing impairment may occur. Controlling the nasal problems, as outlined above using preventers (inhaled steroids), usually allows the middle ear to drain. Decongestants similar to those used to clear the nose may be needed. If middle ear infection occurs, vigorous and prolonged antibiotic treatment is vital to clear up the problem. Sometimes, drainage tubes must be inserted. Good treatment of the underlying problems and control of the middle ear infection will usually prevent permanent injury to the ears and maintain good hearing.

16 Is Your Job Causing Your Asthma?

DURING the past 20 years, asthma has become the most common cause of occupational lung disease, replacing scarring diseases due to inhaled particles and fibres, such as silicosis in sand blasters or miners and asbestosis in shipyard or insulation workers.

The fact that you have developed asthma while at a particular occupation does not necessarily mean that the dust or vapour to which you are exposed at your job is in fact **causing** your problem; it may simply be acting as an irritant "trigger." This is true even if your work is dusty or fume-laden and exposes you to known asthma-causing substances (sensitizers). Asthma in this setting may, however, be caused by exposure to dusts, chemicals, vapours, or fumes that act as "sensitizers." Sensitizers are substances that make you allergic or hypersensitive so that when you encounter them again, you have an unpleasant and sometimes serious reaction to them.

As you may recall from *Chapter 5*, asthma may be either allergic or nonallergic. It is possible that while you are employed in a very dusty occupation, you may develop asthma because of allergy to something totally unrelated to your work, such as pollens in the air during the appropriate season, or cats and house dust mites at home. Alternatively, you may develop the nonallergic type of asthma, which is now thought to follow a severe episode of viral infection of the lung. Nevertheless, if you do develop asthma

while working with chemicals (e.g., toluene diisocyanate in polyurethane), in a foundry or in a very dusty occupation (e.g., Cedarwood dust), you should ask yourself (and your doctor) whether your job might have **caused** your asthma or whether, by virtue of an irritant effect, it might be making your asthma worse.

You probably remember that in *Chapter 6* we indicated that asthma could be caused and resulting airway inflammation worsened by allergens, or attacks be rapidly triggered by nonspecific irritants such as cold air, paint fumes, car exhaust gases, and perfumes. Any of these and other triggers might also irritate your nose and cause the nasal lining to swell within a few minutes of exposure and to discharge mucus (a condition called *rhinitis*, see *Chapter 15*).

Thus, asthma that develops while you are working at a given occupation could simply be a coincidence and

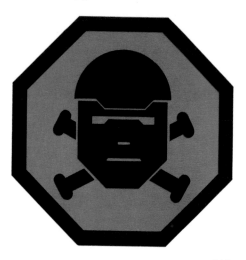

might have occurred no matter what you were doing, but it could be related to your job if you have been exposed to sensitizers and have become sensitized (i.e., allergic). The sensitizers may be well known or as yet undiscovered, especially if you are working with a new chemical process. Finally, gases, fumes, or particles at your job could be acting as nonspecific irritants to cause deterioration of the asthma, which you might have had before or which might have developed related to or unrelated to your job.

It is usually easy to guess that asthma may be job-related under the following circumstances:
1. If the asthma begins within weeks or months of starting a new job.
2. If the asthma regularly and predictably comes on while you are at work or within a few hours after you have finished work.
3. If you seem to improve when you are away from your work, on weekends or especially during holidays, but the asthma returns almost immediately when you resume the same job.
4. If you happen to be working with known sensitizers (see Table 16–1, p. 120).
5. If you work with others, a few of whom seem to be developing similar problems.

Many large industries now employ health and safety staff who can tell you whether or not you are exposed to any known sensitizers, should you begin to experience recurring cough, phlegm production, wheezing, chest tightness, and unusual breathlessness at rest and on exertion. The safety staff can often find out the exact composition of the various substances that you work with and whether any of these substances is known to cause asthma. If you are working with chemical processes that have existed for a long time and that have not in the past been linked to asthma, it is highly unlikely that you will develop the condition when working with such substances. However, asthma that was present when you began to work in that particular occupation might be made worse by almost any volatile chemical substance (remember many substances such as perfumes or household sprays may act as triggers) or by dust particles in high concentrations. If the process that you are working with is relatively new, so that few workers have previously been exposed to the same chemicals, then the asthma that you have developed might signal your unfortunate discovery of a new sensitizing agent.

Of course, the sooner this is investigated and the association between exposure to that particular chemical and asthma is established, the better the situation will be for yourself and many others. Employers may not immediately realize that additional precautions will be necessary when using a particular chemical or chemicals. However, once the sensitizing substances are identified, the appropriate government authorities would hopefully ensure that they are well controlled by isolating the process from the workers or requesting that effective exhaust systems be installed to protect workers. If all else fails the process may need to be changed.

Once you suspect that your asthma symptoms are job related, you should initially discuss the problem with your family doctor, who will provide treatment (see *Chapter 11*) to bring your problem under control. You and the doctor may then wish to report the problem to a body such as the Health and Safety Executive or a workers' compensation board (if there is one), and you should request a referral to a lung specialist who specializes in occupational asthma.

With special tests the respirologist

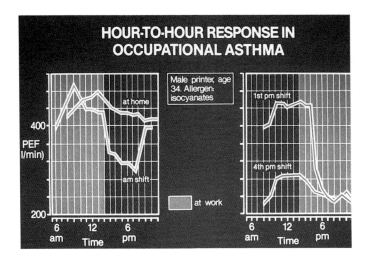

HOUR-TO-HOUR RESPONSE IN OCCUPATIONAL ASTHMA

Male printer, age 34. Allergen: isocyanates

at home

am shift

1st pm shift

4th pm shift

at work

PEF (l/min)

400

200

6 am — 12 — 6 pm — Time

6 am — 12 — 6 pm — Time

can confirm the diagnosis and the association with a chemical sensitizer. If you have, in fact, identified a previously unrecognized sensitizer, the specialist will probably publish your case (or a series of cases if some of your co-workers also have the same problem). This will make sure that the information is disseminated worldwide, thus helping others.

TESTING FOR OCCUPATIONAL ASTHMA

Testing an individual who may have occupational asthma is a painstaking and often prolonged task that requires the full cooperation of the patient and much tenacity on the part of the doctor, so that the association between the occupational exposure and the individual's asthma can be proved beyond reasonable doubt. Such testing may involve frequent measurements of the peak flow rate (see *Chapter 9*) while you are at work, as well as before and after work, on weekends, and during holidays, to find out if the peak flow falls when you are at work or within a few hours of leaving the job. Job-related asthma often starts gradually at the beginning of the work week, and then gets progressively worse as

the week goes on, only to improve again on the weekend or when you go on holidays. This provides important evidence that a problem related to your job exists.

However, often this is not sufficient to establish whether your occupation is actually **causing** your asthma, or whether it is simply acting as a non-specific factor to make your irritable airways go into spasm. In the simplest and most obvious cases, asthma may be present only during the work week, clear up greatly on weekends or when you are on holidays, and disappear if your holiday lasts for 2 to 4 weeks, only to recur immediately or shortly after you return to work.

Unfortunately, the problem is not always this straightforward, because the inflammation that is at the basis of your asthma may settle down only slowly when you are away from work, so that a weekend is not nearly long enough for the asthma to clear up and so establish the association. Also, if you are an allergic person and you go on vacation at a time when you are exposed to substances (e.g., grass pollen) to which you may be allergic, the process initiated at work might be made worse by the allergen exposure.

115

Thus, it will be impossible for you or your doctor to tell to what extent your job may be causing or increasing your asthma.

The next step in establishing the association between your asthma symptoms and your work exposure is to confirm that you do, in fact, have one of the most characteristic features of asthma, namely hyperreactive or "twitchy" airways (a reflection of the fact that airways are inflamed, as you discovered in *Chapter 5*). The test that establishes this in a reliable way (that is, the test is fairly specific for asthma and is also sensitive in excluding non-asthmatics) is called the *inhalation challenge test*. This test can be either specific, that is, you are exposed to, or "challenged" with, a substance to which your doctor believes you to be sensitised (allergic); or nonspecific, that is, you are challenged by inhaling a chemical substance such as histamine (to which asthmatic air passages show an increased reaction) in graded concentrations, starting with a tiny dose and gradually increasing the dose until there is a small reduction in the peak flow rate or the 1 second forced expired volume test (see *Chapter 9*).

The nonspecific test (with the histamine) tells whether you have *nonspecific hyperresponsiveness* — a characteristic of virtually all asthmatics. The specific challenge test (with the allergen or sensitizing chemical to which you may be reacting at work) is used to try to establish exactly what is causing your problem. If you are shown to have nonspecific (histamine, or other triggers) hyperresponsiveness but no specific reaction to the chemicals at work, your doctor would conclude that you do have asthma, but it is not **caused** by the suspect chemicals or dusts at work. The fact that you have problems while you are at work is simply a coincidence — you happened to develop asthma, as many adults

can, **while** you were working at that particular job and not as a **result** of the particular occupation in which you are engaged.

Ideally, the testing is carried out in a manner that doctors call "double blind." That is, you are asked to inhale either the test substance or a dummy resembling the test substance in appearance, smell, and/or taste (placebo) but does not contain the specific chemical or dust for which you are being tested. This is done under circumstances in which neither you nor the doctor carrying out the test knows which of these is being given on any given day. By doing the test in this way, on several occasions, it should be possible to establish clearly whether or not you are sensitive to a questionable substance at work, thus proving beyond any reasonable doubt cause and effect.

MANAGING OCCUPATIONAL ASTHMA

If you have asthma because of work exposure, every possible effort should be made to transfer you to a job that does not contain the substance to which you are sensitive (even in minute amounts). This should be done even if your symptoms can be reasonably well controlled with medication. Not only is your asthma likely to continue while you are exposed to the substance, but the longer the exposure lasts, the more likely it is that the asthma will continue indefinitely after the exposure is stopped.

So, if you develop asthma while engaged in a particular occupation, it is extremely important that you quickly establish whether an association might exist. You should seek appropriate professional help, after which prompt testing should be done to establish whether in fact a relationship exists to your job. If an association is shown to exist, you should make every

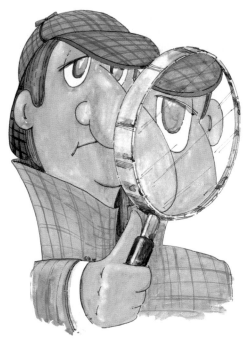

WHAT JOBS ARE LINKED TO ASTHMA?

Table 16–1 (p. 120) contains a partial list of the occupations and/or chemicals known to cause asthma. However, if your occupational exposure is not on the list, this does **not** mean that it could not be causing your problem. Approximately 24,000 new chemicals are introduced to the workplace each year, and some of these will inevitably turn out to be sensitizers.

You shouldn't forget your hobbies either since many of us spend almost as much time at these activities as we do at our jobs, and sensitizers may be present.

Fumes from glues, solvents and soldering fluxes can all cause asthma symptoms.

BE YOUR OWN DETECTIVE!

You are increasingly suspicious that the asthma you developed while at a certain job is actually caused by the job and is not just a coincidence. How are you to proceed? First of all, carry a little diary with you to note down your

effort to change your occupation or to completely eliminate the exposure, in the hope that the asthma will gradually disappear. Remember, the longer you continue your exposure to sensitizers, the less likely you are to be "cured" when exposure ceases.

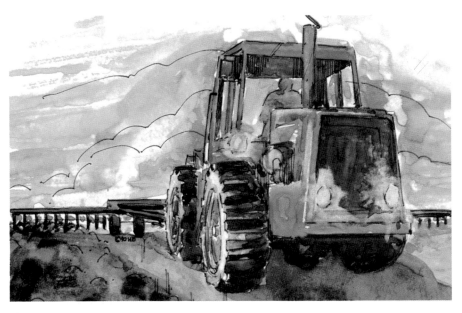

symptoms and their severity (use a scale of 0=no symptoms, 1+=mild, 2+=moderate, 3+=severe). Do this over a period of several weeks to see if your symptoms are generally worse during the work week, tend to improve on the weekend, and seem to gradually clear completely or almost completely the longer you are away from work during vacation.

Once you have established that there appears to be a relationship between your work and the severity of your asthma (and/or nasal) symptoms, find out exactly what substances you may be exposed to at work (or in the pursuit of your hobby, if you think that may be the problem). Manufacturers are usually required to provide a list of the substances contained within a brand name product, but you may have to go back to the original packaging to find it. Failing that, you can contact the manufacturer, the appropriate government department (Department of Health, Ministry of Labour, Community Services) or, in larger industries, the health and safety officer of your union.

The kinds of things that you should be looking for include allergenic proteins, particularly animal skin, birds, glue, sea animals, or sea food, and insects such as weevils or mites in grain. Certain plant proteins such as cereal grains, flour, green coffee, linseed, tobacco leaf, tea, vegetable enzymes, and vegetable gums may also be sensitizers.

In the chemical industry, the major problems are found in the manufacture of plastics (phthalic anhydride); the manufacture or use of epoxy resins (trimellitic anhydride); platinum refining (ammonium tetrachloroplatinate); the dyeing industry; automobile manufacture; paint, varnish, and foundry core makers; and the production or foaming of polyurethane (diisocyanates). Moulds may be a problem in cheese production and in the phar-

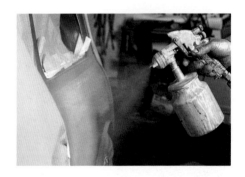

maceutical industry (e.g., penicillin, psyllium). Beauticians may develop asthma because of chemicals such as ethylenediamine, or preexisting asthma may be made worse by petroleum distillates such as perfumes and hairsprays.

Exposure to metal salts such as nickel, chromium, aluminum, and vanadium in metal plating industries, cement manufacture, leather tanning, metal refining, or smelting may cause asthma. Formalin in high concentrations may also cause asthma (although not in the usual concentrations found in homes, even if the insulation is urea formaldehyde foam insulation).

A more complete list of known asthma-producing substances and the associated occupations is found in Table 16–1. This list is incomplete, partly because some of the chemical substances currently in industry have not yet been identified as agents that can produce asthma, and partly because new chemicals are being introduced into the workplace on a daily basis, some of which will doubtless turn out to be asthma-causing agents. The jobs that most commonly predispose to asthma include animal handling in pet shops or laboratories (rats, hamsters, cats, mice, birds), electronics industry work, grain handling, baking, manufacturing of catalytic converters for cars, polyurethane shoe sole and varnish work, woodworking, and farming.

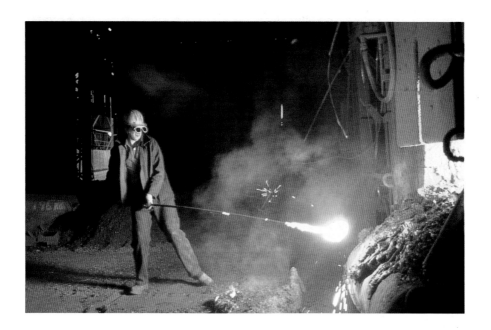

To sum up: it is clear that many occupations are associated with the possibility of developing asthma. Fortunately, in most occupations, even if you are intensely exposed to some of these sensitizers, the chance of your actually developing asthma is relatively small (perhaps 5 to 10 percent). However, this is not true in industries involving exposure to platinum salts where, with time, most of the workers will become sensitized. For this reason, most of these industries now enclose such processes and make sure that they are safely exhausted by using negative-pressure rooms. They also provide scuba-like equipment or spacesuits for people having to work in or service such areas.

Keep in mind that it is not necessary for **you yourself** to actually be **working** with these chemicals in order for you to develop asthma because of them. It may be sufficient for you to be working in a building where such chemicals are being released if you share the same air, and if exhaust systems for those chemicals are less

than 100 percent efficient, as is usually the case. This is because minute amounts of the chemical (a few parts per billion) may be sufficient to cause sensitization and give you ongoing asthma. In England a number of workers developed asthma simply because their factory's air intake was beside the exhaust outlet of a neighbouring factory where toluene diisocyanate was used to produce polyurethane foam shoe soles.

Another unfortunate fact about occupational asthma is that if you remain exposed for more than a short period of time after the asthma has started, the condition may become permanent, even if you subsequently **leave that job and are no longer exposed to that chemical!** This makes it essential that occupational asthma be noticed quickly, identified for what it is, and that you be removed from the hazard or, alternatively, that the hazardous substance be exhausted in such a way that you are no longer exposed to it (even in very small amounts).

TABLE 16-1 OCCUPATIONS ASSOCIATED WITH OCCUPATIONAL ASTHMA

Industry/Occupation	Agent
Farmers	Horses, cattle, pigs, moulds, grain weevils
Animal handlers (laboratory, workers, veterinary, surgeons)	Rat, mouse, rabbit, guinea pig
Bakers	Wheat, rye, buckwheat
Crab processors	Crab
Detergent industry	Biological enzymes
Appliance manufacturing (polyurethane foam insulation)	Isocyanates
Automobile spray painting	Isocyanates
Electronics	Rosin, thallium anhydride
Foundries (mould makers)	Isocyanates, furans
Lumber (carpentry, sawmill)	Western red cedar
Metal plating	Nickel, chromium
Pharmaceuticals	Psyllium, antibiotics
Plastics, epoxy resins	Anhydrides
Platinum refining	Platinum salts

TREATMENT OF OCCUPATIONAL ASTHMA

The single most important way to treat this kind of asthma once it has been **proven** that it is occupation-related is to remove yourself from the exposure as rapidly and completely as possible. As soon as you **suspect** that the asthma is related to your work environment, you should tell your supervisor, notify the health and safety officer of your union. Fortunately, occupational asthma usually responds to the same sorts of treatments as asthma caused by allergens or the non-allergic forms of asthma. Asthma treatment is explained in detail in *Chapter 11*.

A Note of Caution: Do not leave your job until an association has been established, since if it is subsequently shown that your asthma is not job related you may have left a job that you were skilled at and enjoyed, and you would not be eligible for compensation.

17 Asthma and Pregnancy

PREGNANCY is inevitably a time of great physical and emotional stress. This is especially true if you have asthma, particularly if the asthma is not well controlled. Poor asthma control leads to sleeplessness and increased exhaustion and could lead to severe attacks that could place your life and that of the foetus at risk. So good control should be the goal, to make sure that you will feel your very best at this very important time in the lives of you and your baby.

TAKING MEDICATION? THINK TWICE!

You should naturally be careful about any medications you take during your pregnancy, particularly during the first 3 months, when the organs of the baby are being formed. Almost everyone now knows that some medications or indeed any chemical substances taken into your baby may interfere with normal development of the unborn baby and so should be avoided whenever possible. These, of course, include over-the-counter medicines from drug stores, tobacco smoked or chewed, marijuana, cocaine, heroin, alcohol, and others too numerous to mention.

IN PREGNANCY, ASTHMA CONTROL IS MORE IMPORTANT THAN EVER

If you are asthmatic, a most important consideration should be good control of the asthma with medications that are safe for both you and your foetus. This will help avoid severe attacks, which may cause low levels of oxygen in your blood and which could also

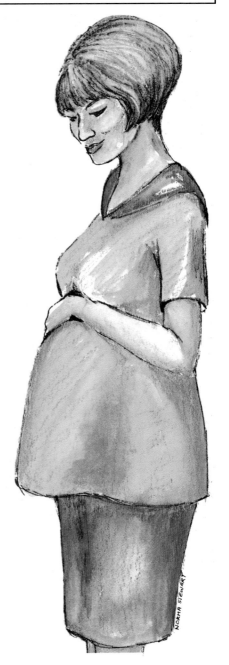

injure the baby. Fortunately, most of the currently used, really effective asthma medications have **not** been associated with birth defects or any other harmful effects on your developing baby. Table 17–1 (p. 125) lists virtually all classes of medication used in patients with asthma and their relative safety during pregnancy.

ASTHMA TREATMENT DURING PREGNANCY

AVOIDANCE

The best way to stay free of asthma and at the same time reduce the need to take medications is to avoid the things that you know cause asthma attacks. For example, if you are allergic to cats or dogs you should, more than at any other time, remove such pets from your environment and, if possible, avoid visiting people that have such animals. During the pollen season, avoidance can be accomplished by staying indoors when pollen counts are highest, by means of air-conditioned bedrooms and cars, and by avoiding the countryside. Non-specific irritants such as tobacco or any other kind of smoke, strong smelling chemicals, and cold air exposure should also be avoided if these cause asthma to flare up.

However, this does **not** mean that you should avoid skiing or social situations where you may encounter perfumes and a moderate amount of secondhand smoke. If you have asthma attacks requiring extra bronchodilator puffs under these conditions, your asthma is **out of control** and requires reassessment by your doctor, who will improve the controlling treatment (see *Chapter 11*). However, before calling your doctor, make sure that you are taking **all** medications in the prescribed doses and that you are using your inhalers properly.

Studies have shown that desensitization injections can continue during your pregnancy as long as you do not develop local or widespread reactions. Bee sting venom treatment can also continue safely. Allergy skin tests are occasionally associated with widespread reactions, so you should probably avoid getting these done while you are pregnant.

MEDICATIONS DURING PREGNANCY

As indicated above, a minimum of all kinds of medication is the ideal that should be aimed at during the first 3 months of pregnancy. However, in mothers-to-be with asthma, **all** asthma-controlling medications **must be continued** because the low oxygen levels associated with a severe attack could be harmful to the unborn baby. The asthma medications now commonly used, with very rare exceptions, have been shown to be extremely safe (see Table 17–1).

ASTHMA MAY BE EASIER TO CONTROL DURING PREGNANCY

During pregnancy, particularly in the middle and final three-month periods (trimesters), about two-thirds of women notice that their asthma actually improves, whereas about one-third of women experience worsening of their asthma. Recent studies have suggested that the improvement is probably related to reduced inflammation in the air passages due to the same natural hormones that prevent rejection of the placenta (the placenta is the baby's tissues and would be rejected like a kidney transplant were it not for these hormones).

WHY DOES ASTHMA GET WORSE IN SOME PREGNANT WOMEN?

The cause of asthma deterioration in one-third of women is not known. It may be partly caused by regurgitation of acid into the oesophagus (or gullet, which connects the mouth to the stomach), and the back of the throat, particularly when you are asleep. Small amounts of acid may then spill over into the windpipe and the lungs. This may cause irritation of the lining of the air passages, leading to deterioration of the asthma. Other factors that may make the effects of inadequately controlled asthma worse include emotional and physical stress and the increasing size of the abdomen associated with the baby's development, which tends to push the diaphragm upwards and contributes to shortness of breath on physical activity, bending over or lying down.

During pregnancy, the treatments used to control asthma are no different from those needed when you are not pregnant. Wherever possible, use the aerosol form of bronchodilators, which give very low blood levels, (cromoglycate), or inhaled steroids — these medications are both effective and safe. Medications in the form of tablets, which are in any case less effective than sprays, should be avoided, if possible. Tablets are more likely to cause side effects to you and your unborn baby. Although large doses of cortisone medications given as tablets or injections (not if given by aerosol in appropriate doses) for prolonged periods of time (months or years) may cause you potential problems (see *Chapter 11*), your foetus should be little affected.

Given the powerful and safe inhaled steroids that are available, it is unlikely that you would need steroid tablets long term since most asthma can nowadays be controlled entirely by the use of aerosols. Even if you do need steroid tablets to control your obviously severe asthma, the effect on the baby is usually insignificant, although it has been suggested, but not proven, that there might be a slightly increased incidence of cleft palate and spinal abnormalities in the baby if the mother needs large and ongoing doses of steroids (prednisolone) tablets.

BREAST-FEEDING

If you are using inhaled treatments, these should not get into the breast milk in sufficient amounts that the baby will be affected. The tablet forms of bronchodilator treatment will get into the milk, and your baby may develop minor symptoms such as restlessness or irritability. There is much debate about the possible benefit of breast-feeding for at least 3 to 6 months for the prevention of allergy later in your child's life. On the other hand, it has also been suggested that eating certain foods such as shellfish and peanuts while breast-feeding might actually predispose the baby to allergies later. Perhaps the best compromise is to breast-feed for 6 months or more while avoiding these foods.

In moderate doses, there is little potential harm to the nursing infant from steroids, although this may not be the case if very large doses of pred-

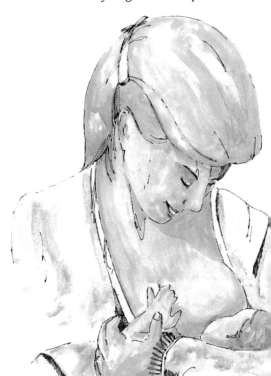

nisolone/methylprednisolone are required for many weeks or months during severe asthma flare-ups. Under these conditions, your doctor may advise you to stop breast-feeding. If steroid tablets have to be used, your doctor can advise on the medication which will protect the baby from side effects.

If antibiotics are necessary during pregnancy, most of them can be used and are perfectly safe. Exceptions to this are the following:

1. Tetracycline antibiotics, which will mottle the teeth of the baby
2. Co-trimoxazole (Septrin, Bactrim), an antibiotic that blocks the action of an important vitamin (folic acid), which is needed for normal development of the baby.
3. Quinolone antibiotics (Norfloxacin, Ciprofloxacin) — these may interfere with cartilage development in beagle dogs but not other animals. The possible effect in humans is not yet certain.

In addition, codeine should be avoided during the first 3 months of pregnancy because there is suspicion that it can cause abnormalities of development in the baby. However, a similar substance frequently found in cough medicines, dextromethorphan, appears to be safe.

SOME GENERAL FACTS ABOUT ASTHMA AND PREGNANCY

Studies have shown that babies of asthmatic mothers have a greater risk of being born prematurely and, even if not premature, their birth weight tends to be lower than average. On the other hand, spontaneous abortions and birth defects are **not** increased.

All pregnant women who smoke should discontinue the habit at once because of the well-known harmful effects on both the mother and the foetus. This is especially true of the smoking asthmatic, who runs a greatly increased risk of a severe asthma attack at some time in the pregnancy. This could seriously reduce the oxygen supply to the unborn baby, particularly if the blood of the foetus already contains a large amount of carbon monoxide gas from cigarette smoke. This reduces the ability of the blood to carry life-giving oxygen from the lungs to the cells in all parts of the body.

During your pregnancy, you should **always** take the medication prescribed to **control your asthma** by your doctor to **avoid severe asthma attacks**. Frequent supervision by your doctor is important in order to adjust the medications you require to keep you free of symptoms.

NOSE PROBLEMS

During pregnancy, many women have problems with stuffiness and plugging of their noses and over-production of mucus from the nose, whether they are asthmatic or not. This problem may be even greater in patients with asthma. The effects on the nose, particularly the congestion, are probably caused by the generalized congestion of blood vessels throughout the body during pregnancy. Certain normal hormonal and nervous system effects may make matters even worse. Associated with the nasal problems may be loss of the sense of smell; sleeping with the mouth open at night, resulting in a very dry mouth in the morning; and congestion and stuffiness of the ears because of swelling of the eustachian tube, which normally drains the middle ear. This congestion may lead to fluid build-up in the middle ear region, which may temporarily reduce your hearing.

Although you may be able to put up with the nasal stuffiness fairly well if the symptoms are mild, you should know that a great deal can be done about the condition. If the stuffiness is

TABLE 17-1 SAFETY OF DRUGS USED TO TREAT ASTHMA AND RHINITIS DURING PREGNANCY

	Considered Safe	Probably Safe	Unknown	Avoid
Inhaled Medications				
Corticosteroid (aerosol)				
Becotide, Becloforte,	X			
Pulmicort	X			
Flixotide		X		
Anticholinergic				
Atrovent, Oxivent (aerosol)		X		
Rinatec (nasal spray)		X		
Cromoglycates (aerosol)				
Intal	X			
Nedocromil	X			
Beta-Agonists (aerosol)		X		
Bricanyl, Ventolin, Berotec,		X		
Tablets				
Steroids				
Prednisone/Prednisolone		X		
Methylprednisolone		X		
Theophylline (many brands,		X		
e.g., Theo-Dur,		X		
Phyllocontin,		X		
Choledyl, Nuelin)		X		
Immunotherapy				
Allergy injections (if you are already taking these)		X		
Allergy skin tests			X	
Antibiotics				
Tetracycline/co-trimoxazole				X
Penicillin/cephalosporins	X			
Ciprofloxacin, Norfloxacin			X	
Cough and Pain Medication				
Codeine				X
Dextromethorphan	X			
Acetaminophen	X			
Aspirin				X
Antihistamines				
Piriton (chlorpheniramine)		X		
Triludan, Teldane (terfenadine)			X	
Hismanal (astemizole)			X	
Zaditen (ketotifen)			X	
Claritin, Claratyne (loratadine)			X	

Note: Inhaled medications are always much safer than pills or injections!

bothersome, it can usually be treated effectively. If the problem occurs only occasionally, then a nasal spray such as oxymetazoline hydrochloride (Otrivin) used sparingly may be sufficient. However, this medication should not be used regularly for more than a week because it may·cause permanent damage to the lining of your nose, leading to rebound swelling — a cycle that may be hard to break later. Other treatments include a nasal spray of cromoglycate (Rynacrom®) or steroids (Beconase®, Vancenase®, Rhinocort). Some pregnant women are helped by a nasal spray of an anticholinergic agent (Rinatec®). Sometimes, a special salt water spray can be helpful.

LABOUR AND DELIVERY

With close supervision, your asthma should be under good control when you go into labour. If this is the case, you should have no difficulty whatsoever, and you should simply go on taking the same medications that you were taking before labour began. These medications should be continued after the baby has been delivered.

If you were one of the fortunate two-thirds of women whose asthma improved during the pregnancy, and you were able to greatly reduce your medication, you will probably have in-creased medication needs within a few hours or days after the baby has been delivered. We suggest that you be prepared to resume the same doses of medication after delivery that were needed to control your asthma before your pregnancy and during the first 3 months.

If your asthma is not under good control when you go into labour, you should not wait at home until your labour is far advanced and the baby is ready for delivery. Instead, you should go to the hospital (or contact your doctor) as soon as contractions begin. This may give your doctor (and, if necessary, the lung specialist) a chance to bring the asthma under really good control before labour is advanced. This avoids subjecting the baby to low oxygen levels during delivery.

To summarize, during pregnancy you, the pregnant asthmatic, should avoid those things that you know cause irritation or flare-ups of the asthma, just as you have always done but even more rigorously. You should take all of the medications that your doctor has prescribed to keep the asthma under excellent control so that you will not have flare-ups of asthma during pregnancy or delivery. This will help to ensure that you will be well and deliver a normal, healthy baby.

18 Can Asthma Be Inherited?

A QUESTION that is commonly asked, particularly by pregnant women and by parents of young children who themselves have asthma, is "can my child inherit my asthma?" It is well known that the tendency to develop allergies can be inherited and sometimes is. Typically children, some of whom later develop allergic inflammation of the nose or airways (rhinitis or asthma) have an inflammatory skin condition called *eczema* that begins in infancy and early childhood. This rash is usually seen as an area of roughness and irritation of the skin with itching and sometimes weeping in the skin creases in front of the elbow and behind the knees. Later on, about one-third of these children develop a runny, stuffy, plugged-up nose (allergic rhinitis or hay fever), frequently followed by episodes of sinus or ear infection. About one-fifth of such children may develop asthma.

There are 100,000 human genes, and recently, the single abnormal gene accounting for most of the tendency to develop allergies has been identified. The defective gene has been found in about one out of four people in England. Most of these people had some allergic complaints, and one in twenty had asthma. Understanding the genetic basis for allergy may at some time in the future lead to better treatments. However, the inheritance of asthma is not all that certain. Even with identical twins (who share exactly the same genes), in only about 20 percent will the one twin develop asthma if the other twin is asthmatic. This means that factors in the environment are important in determining whether an individual develops asthma, although the allergic tendency obviously makes it somewhat more likely. The nonallergic form of asthma (see *Chapter 8*) is much less likely to have a genetic basis. Indeed, there is considerable debate about whether this type of asthma is inherited at all.

At present, even if there is a hereditary basis to asthma, not much is known about how this causes the asthmatic condition, so it is not yet possible to use this information to avoid the development of asthma. However, the presence of asthma in a number of blood relatives should alert you to the possibility that your child may have this condition if, during infancy, the child frequently develops nasal plugging, sinus and middle ear infections, episodes of "bronchitis" or "croup" with or without wheezing, or a persistent cough. You should also carefully consider whether under those circumstances, you should acquire family pets such as cats, dogs, hamsters, or birds, since these pets may trigger allergies, leading to nasal problems and/or asthma.

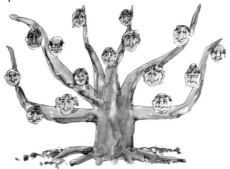

19 Asthma: An "Emotional Problem"?

IR WILLIAM OSLER, one of the greatest physicians of the late nineteenth century (see *Chapter 2*), suggested that asthma was a "neurotic" disease. This idea soon became widespread and continued to have a considerable influence on doctors in their care of asthmatic patients until about fifteen years ago.

Doctors who thought that asthma was a neurotic disease approached treatment by dealing mainly with stress factors related to their patients' home life or work. They had little success, despite the use of psychotherapy, sedatives, hypnosis, and medications aimed at treating anxiety or depression. This is because asthma is not chiefly an emotional disease, although stresses of all kinds may make asthma worse **if it is poorly controlled**. In the same way, running and other exercise may bring on wheezing when asthma is not properly controlled, but we know that exercise is not the **cause** of asthma.

These doctors may have had the cart before the horse when they described a typical asthma personality. People with this so-called "asthma personality" were described as anxious and depressed. This is not surprising, since asthma treatment in those days was ineffective and the disease often prevented those who suffered from it from leading a normal existence.

We know now that asthma is not a neurotic disease in the usual sense, although people with severe and uncontrolled asthma may be anxious and depressed. We also know that if asthma is well controlled, people with this condition have no more emotional problems than those who do not suffer from asthma and are able to live quite normally and to carry on with their lives reasonably well.

In summary, asthma is **not** a neurotic illness, but major emotional stresses will tend to make asthma symptoms worse if the asthma is poorly controlled. However, this is unlikely if the asthma is well controlled using modern treatment methods.

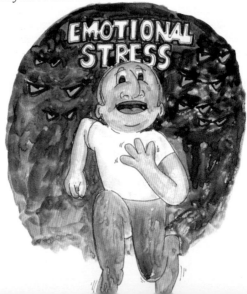

20 Food, Diet, and Asthma

PATIENTS with asthma often wonder whether the food they eat may make their symptoms worse. There is still much uncertainty about diet and asthma, and so confusing advice is often given.

FOOD ALLERGY AND ASTHMA

A true allergic reaction to food is uncommon. Sometimes people have an acute reaction after eating small quantities of certain foods, such as nuts or some types of shellfish. This reaction may start with a tingling sensation in the mouth or on the lips or tightness of the throat, associated with a general flushing. The lips, throat, and tongue may swell, making breathing difficult, and a widespread itchy rash may break out. This reaction may be accompanied by wheezing and, in serious attacks, there may be fainting and collapse. This acute reaction is called *anaphylaxis* and comes on within minutes of eating the particular food. These reactions can be very serious, so the food in question must be carefully avoided in future. This may be difficult, since even minute quantities of the food can trigger an attack.

These attacks must be treated immediately. The most effective treatment is an injection of adrenaline, although an adrenaline inhaler is easier to self-administer and works just as well, provided that a sufficient number of puffs, to the point of trembling and heart palpitations (perhaps 10 to 15 puffs), are taken.

The allergic response to certain foods that comes on more slowly is more difficult to assess. Some people with asthma notice that their symptoms are worse after eating certain foods, such as dairy products or eggs. Sometimes there is a positive skin reaction to an extract of these foods, but frequently skin tests are negative.

Asthma symptoms should improve if the food is excluded from the diet. In the case of common foods like eggs, this is often difficult, since so many of the foods we eat contain eggs. If symptoms do improve with this sort of exclusion diet, it may be worth trying to reintroduce the food again to see

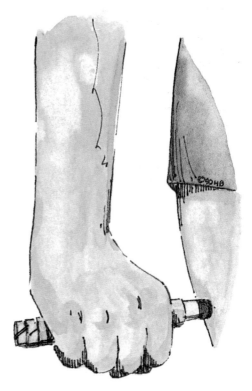

whether it brings on asthma symptoms. The symptoms may develop several hours after eating the food and may be accompanied by other general symptoms such as tiredness, depression, and headache. Obviously, the best advice is to avoid these foods.

The only way to be absolutely sure that a certain food is making asthma worse is to be given the food under circumstances where neither the doctor nor the patient is aware of whether or not the food is being given (double-blind test). This can be done by giving either the food or a dummy (placebo) in a capsule. Such tests are obviously time-consuming and may be misleading, since only small amounts of food can be given in capsules. When these "challenge" studies are done on patients who suspect certain foods of worsening their asthma only a few have a positive result under these controlled circumstances. Perhaps the best advice if you suspect that a certain type of food is making your asthma worse is to try to avoid the food completely for a period of 2 weeks. If your asthma gets better, try the food again and, if it does make your symptoms worse, then avoid that food in future. Thus, you can be your own detective.

In children, food allergies to milk and eggs may disappear as they grow older, so it may be worth trying the offending food again after 6 to 12 months. This does not apply to anaphylactic reactions to foods (especially peanuts and shellfish) — these foods should **not** be "tried" for fear of severe reactions that could be life-threatening.

Since all of the ingredients in packaged foods do not always appear on the label and, for example, some fast foods are fried in peanut oil without your knowing it, you should avoid, and teach your child with anaphylaxis to avoid, all foods not prepared at home. The following case history tragically illustrates this point.

J.S., a 15-year-old boy who had always been very cautious about what he ate because of known peanut anaphylaxis, went to a fast food restaurant with his friends. He was assured by the proprietor that the food he ordered did not contain nuts of any kind. Minutes later, he had a severe anaphylactic reaction. Unfortunately, he did not have his autoinjectable adrenaline syringe or his bronchodilator inhaler (which he was told always to carry) with him. He was dead before he reached the hospital. At the inquest, it was revealed that although the food did not contain nuts, it had been cooked in peanut oil, which is often used for baking and frying because of its lightness and lack of taste.

FOOD AND DRINK ADDITIVES

It has recently been recognized that several of the artificial colourings, flavourings, and preservatives added to food can worsen asthma. It is important to know about the main culprits, since it is possible to avoid them. Food additives now have to be listed on the product label so you can check for them before eating the particular food, and it is now often possible to buy foods that are "preservative free." In Europe, these additives have been given numbers, which have to appear on the packaging. Some of the most troublesome chemicals include the following:

Sulphites and sulphur dioxide (E220, 221, 222, 226, 227) are used as preservatives in food and drink and are commonly found in certain beers and wines (especially sparkling wines), in lettuce, which is often washed in a solution of metabisulphite to keep it looking fresh (particularly in restaurant salad bars), in instant soups, synthetic orange drinks, and cooked meats (e.g., salami).

Tartrazine (E102) is a dye that colours food yellow or orange. It may

130

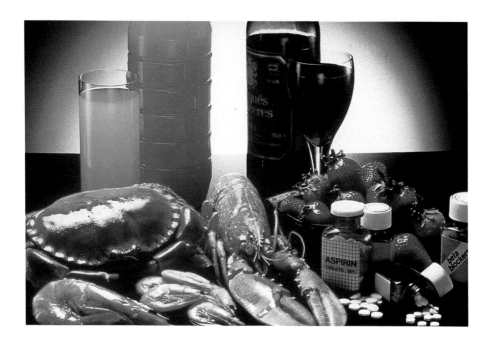

also be used to colour capsules and medicines. It rarely causes asthma symptoms, but when it occurs it does so particularly in children.

Benzoic acid (E210) is used as a preservative and can also be troublesome for asthmatics.

Aspirin and salicylates and related treatments can cause worsening of symptoms in a small proportion of people with asthma (see *Chapter 8*). It has now been recognized that aspirin and related salicylates may occur naturally in certain foods. This may lead to worsening of asthma and may be associated with other symptoms, such as tiredness, mouth ulcers, and bowel disturbances. Foods that contain these chemicals include yeast extract, mushrooms, and chocolate.

Monosodium glutamate (MSG, E621) is added to food as a flavour enhancer. It is found in soy sauce, spices, stock cubes, crisps, potato chips, bacon, hamburgers, and packaged soups. It is used excessively in some Chinese restaurants. Some people react to large doses of MSG with symptoms of sweating, flushing, numbness of the chest, and faintness, while some people with asthma may develop an attack of wheezing that may begin several hours after the meal ("Chinese restaurant asthma syndrome").

SPECIAL DIETS

You may have read about a number of diets that claim to make asthma better. These claims are false, and in general, such diets cannot be recommended. However, if you are overweight, it is sensible to lose weight, since being too heavy imposes an extra demand on your breathing capacity.

If you find that some kinds of food make your asthma worse, these are best avoided. For the reasons discussed earlier, it is also sensible to avoid additives in food wherever possible. If you find that you react to particular additives such as sulphites, then check the contents of any packaged food you eat.

131

Lately, there has been much interest in whether animal fats should be avoided by people with asthma. Some studies have shown that substituting fish oil for animal fat leads to reduced production of some of the chemicals involved in asthmatic inflammation. The Inuit, who have a diet that is rich in fish, do not seem to have much asthma. However, recent trials of such diets in asthmatic patients, who were given fish oil in the form of capsules, did not show any convincing improvement in their asthma. Perhaps this is because it is not possible to give enough fish oil easily or because the theory is wrong. In any case, such diets cannot be recommended as a way of improving asthma.

Thus, no special diet is particularly useful in asthma, but you should look out for any types of food or drink that make your asthma worse, try to identify the culprit, and then avoid this substance whenever possible.

21 Alternative Therapies

YOU probably have heard of several so-called "alternative" therapies for asthma. These are treatments that are not conventional and are usually given by nonmedical people. Most of these "treatments" do not help asthma and are often very expensive. However, people are sometimes tempted to try alternative therapy, which is often advertised by means of testimonials as having great benefit. People always hope that this will provide a "cure" and allow them to stop their asthma treatments.

It should be stressed that these treatments have no proven benefit when tested in proper clinical trials, although there may appear to be some improvement at first because of the "placebo" effect, since suggestion may, for a short time, improve asthma symptoms.

HYPNOSIS

Hypnosis has been studied in several experimental trials in various types of asthma. Although none of the trials have shown a striking improvement, some individual patients seem to respond to this form of treatment. Thus hypnosis may occasionally be helpful, most often in people for whom stress is a major factor.

ACUPUNCTURE

There has recently been a trend for using acupuncture to treat a variety of diseases. Some studies have found that acupuncture reduced wheezing after exercise and in some other inhaled challenges, but the effects are small. In the most carefully conducted study, no benefit could be shown in asthma symptoms over a 4-week period.

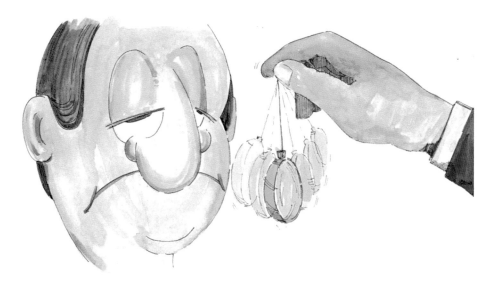

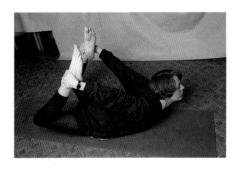

Yoga

Yoga, which has been used in India for centuries to treat many ailments, may be useful in relaxing people with asthma when stress is a particular problem.

Physical Training

Physical training and exercise programmes have been claimed to improve asthma control, particularly in children. There is no concrete evidence to support this idea, but people with asthma (like anyone else) often feel better after regular exercise, which should therefore be encouraged. Children should be encouraged to participate in all sports and should have suitable treatment to prevent the development of wheezing during exercise. Swimming is particularly suitable for asthmatics.

Homoeopathy

Homoeopathic preparations are available for the treatment of asthma, but these have not been tested in properly conducted trials. The scientific basis for homoeopathy is **extremely doubtful**, since it involves diluting the medicinal substance until almost none of it is left.

Negative Ion Generators

Negatively-charged air ions have been claimed to improve asthma, and therefore small machines (like a fan heater) that generate negative ions (ionizers) have been advertised as a help for asthmatics. In a carefully controlled, 6-month study no benefit whatsoever was shown in asthma symptoms. These machines cannot be recommended as an asthma treatment because they are useless and can be expensive.

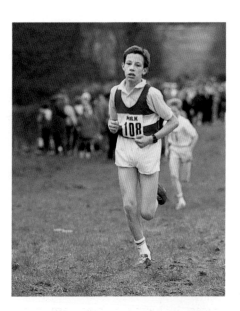

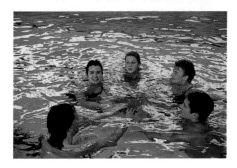

SURGERY

Strangely enough, certain surgical techniques have been used to treat asthma. These include cutting the nerves to the lung or cutting out small glands in the neck, which sense oxygen levels in the blood. These operations have never been tested properly and are probably worthless. Since they are not without risk, they cannot be recommended. Fortunately, surgery for asthma is hardly ever performed today.

BREATHING EXERCISES AND BIOFEEDBACK

Breathing exercises and biofeedback may be useful in preventing a panic reaction to severe asthma attacks. Controlled breathing through pursed lips can help to relieve the symptoms of asthma during an attack. However, there is no evidence that breathing exercises "strengthen the lungs" against asthma, nor that biofeedback does anything but help asthmatics to put up with their symptoms. Above all, these methods should not be considered a substitute for modern asthma treatment.

CLINICAL ECOLOGY

Some people believe that many diseases, including asthma, are caused by the breathing in and eating of even minute amounts of supposedly harmful chemical substances in the environment, and that the only treatment is to completely avoid contact with these substances, by strict diets and sometimes by living in a "bubble" with a supply of purified air. There is no reasonable support for these views. The diets often lead to severe malnutrition and weight loss, and the isolation is extremely stressful.

Lately, much media attention has been given to the so-called yeast (*Candida*) disease, said to be caused by the presence of this common fungus in the intestines. Some clinical ecologists suggest that such conditions result from "immune dysregulation," but they cannot demonstrate that this actually occurs. Nevertheless, a number of illogical, unscientific, and usually expensive treatments have been devised for this non-disease. Usually such treatments (like hypnotherapy, laser treatments, etc.) are given credence by testimonials from supposedly satisfied patients. Since the dummy treatment (i.e., placebo) effect in research trials may be as high as 30 percent of patients in the study, it is not surprising that some people may feel better for a while, no matter what they are given to "treat" their condition.

In fact, such implausible theories and treatments have most of the characteristics of religious cults, so that the believers accept the unproven word of an authority figure (the clinical ecologist). These believers become disciples and are a source for referrals, fund-raising and political action to have the fees funded through a national health service. The patient is promised that they will be "cured" if they follow a tightly controlled programme. However, failure to recover does not usually lead to discarding of the beliefs, because these are necessary to the patient's "need to be sick." Those who do not improve, or exhaust their finances, are often ignored or rejected, resulting in desperate, depressed, and hopeless individuals.

Bogus allergy tests are often linked to this form of medicine. Analysis of a few hairs has been claimed to predict the various things that are causing asthma, so that the current diet and "treatment" can be worked out. These methods, when checked scientifically, have been found to be fraudulent and therefore should be avoided.

CHIROPRACTIC TECHNIQUES

There is no basis whatever for the application of chiropractic techniques to the care of people with asthma.

THE DANGERS OF "ALTERNATIVE" THERAPY

None of these "alternative" treatments have been shown to have any real benefit in treating asthma. On the other hand, few of these therapies are actually harmful, and some (e.g., hypnosis, yoga) may be helpful in patients where stress is a major trigger for asthma. The main danger of these therapies is that they may stop you from taking effective scientifically based asthma treatment, which will almost always work, if taken in adequate doses. As a result, you may end up with asthma that is not well controlled. Taking alternative treatments may also delay seeking informed medical advice. Therefore, we recommend that, **if** you wish to use an alternative therapy, **the normal treatment for asthma must not be stopped** (there is **no** evidence that any of the alternative treatments discussed here are able to reduce the doses of conventional asthma treatments, such as the number of inhaler puffs needed). Furthermore, if you wish to try alternative treatments **in addition** to your regular medication, let your doctor know.

22 Asthma Management – Present and Future

WHILE curing asthma is the ultimate goal of present research, it seems unlikely that this "utopia" can be achieved in the foreseeable future. However, since you have read the previous chapters, you now know that most people with asthma can lead almost completely normal lives provided that, with their doctor's help, they follow some straightforward treatment principles.

You are the most important part of the health care team because, even with the best advice in the world, no good will come of it unless you undertake the necessary self care to achieve an excellent result.

You can do your part by:

1. Removing as many of the known or suspected causes of your condition from your environment as you possibly can. These include allergens such as cats, house dust, mites, pollens, cigarette smoking (including other people's smoke), relevant occupational dusts, fumes, and volatile chemicals, as well as certain drugs that you may be taking for other conditions that may have a harmful effect.
2. Scrupulously following the advice of your doctor to keep the asthma under control. This means taking the preventative medications regularly and using the relievers as needed.
3. Initiating effective treatment to correct deterioration before you get into serious difficulty. Sometimes symptoms will tell you that you are

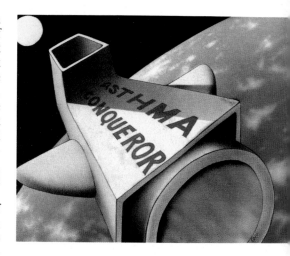

getting worse, while at other times the clue will be that you need more bronchodilator puffs than usual. If you seem to get into serious difficulty without advance warning, you should regularly measure the peak flow, which may alert you to the need to increase the preventer medications before you get into serious difficulty.

4. Arranging with your doctor for regular follow-up visits to make sure that the asthma remains under control and to see to it that you have the advantage of new treatments as they become available.

NEW AND IMPROVED TREATMENTS

Ongoing research has greatly improved our understanding of how inflammation is produced in the airways, leading to the features of the disease we call asthma. Better treatments should eventually become available to counteract the effects of the inflammatory substances that are poured out by injured airway cells in allergic and nonallergic asthma.

Although no dramatically new treatments are likely to be introduced within the next 3 to 5 years, greatly improved variations of present treatments will almost certainly become available in the near future.

BRONCHODILATORS

The most interesting recent developments are new bronchodilator aerosol medicines called salmeterol and formoterol. These act for over 12 hours and will probably replace the current reliever medications such as salbutamol, which only act for 3 to 6 hours. Such long-acting bronchodilators are of particular benefit to otherwise well-controlled asthmatics who still sometimes wake up at night or have chest tightness when they wake up in the morning. They also provide all-day relief from cold air or exercise-related breathlessness.

New, longer-acting, anticholinergic medications (oxitropium bromide) are already available, and even longer acting drugs are under development.

BLOCKERS OF NATURAL CHEMICAL MEDIATORS

In the past few years, asthma research has shown us that the inflammatory reaction causes the release of a great many natural chemicals in our bodies. Some of these chemicals cause narrowing of airways and account for the various features of inflammation, while others counteract their effects and so reduce the amount of inflammation or open up the airways. If we can block the effects of the substances that cause inflammation and bronchoconstriction or increase the natural production of the substances that counteract inflammation, we should be able to develop important new treatments to control asthma and prevent attacks. This research is still in an early stage, and the introduction of these agents for treating asthma is still at least several years away.

INHALED STEROIDS

As you know from *Chapters 10* and *11*, inhaled steroids have been one of the greatest advances in asthma treatment. The presently available steroid aerosols provide excellent control of the inflammation underlying asthma in the majority of people with the disease when these medications are used regularly. They also cause few side effects, which are in any case fairly minor. This ratio of beneficial effects to side effects can be further improved by always inhaling the steroid puffs through an accessory device, preferably one with a valve, such as the Volumatic® or Nebuhaler®. It is likely that during the next 3 to 5 years, improved and more compact accessory devices will be available for use with metered dose inhalers, while multi-dose powder inhalers will become more widespread, thus making asthma treatment safer and more convenient. It is likely that a substitute will be found for the environmentally unfriendly chlorofluorocarbons (pressurization chemicals used in aerosol sprays). This is an important issue because, no matter how effective the powder inhalers are, they may not be able to replace pressurized metered dose inhalers completely, particularly in children under the age of 3 or 4 and in people having severe attacks of asthma. However, compared with Freons used in industry (in refrigeration for example), medical applications use less than 1 percent of the total, making it unlikely that metered dose inhalers are having much effect on the earth's ozone layer.

Even safer inhaled steroids include budesonide (Pulmicort) and the recently introduced fluticasone (Flixotide). These inhaled steroids are even less likely to give rise to side effects and are of particular value in treating children.

ASTHMA MONITORING

Over the next 10 years, it is likely that more and more asthma patients will measure their own peak flow rate. This will be done to make certain that the treatment is controlling the inflammation as effectively as possible, which should result in normally **functioning** lungs, rather than simply suppressing the symptoms. In this way, asthmatics will be able to modify their treatment and so will be able to take care of themselves on a day-to-day basis in the same way as patients with high blood pressure or diabetes. It is important to remember that really good asthma control will probably prevent permanent injury to the air passages.

IMMUNOTHERAPY

During the next 10 years, asthma injection treatment will probably be used less because this form of treatment is not very effective in most asthmatics, while other approaches to treatment are steadily improving. New and safer forms of immunotherapy are now being developed.

ASTHMA TABLETS

Tablets containing theophylline will be used much less frequently during the next 10 years as even better aerosol treatments are introduced. The tablets provide much less benefit than sprays and unfortunately may cause many side effects.

ANTIHISTAMINE TABLETS

A number of antihistamine medications are currently used for asthma treatment. These have not been very effective because histamine is not the only chemical agent underlying inflammation, and therefore blocking histamine alone would be expected to have only a modest effect, at best. It is not likely that this class of compounds will have an important role to play in the care of asthmatic patients in the future.

CURING ASTHMA: THE ULTIMATE GOAL

A cure for asthma is the ideal to which all doctors and research scientists in this field are dedicated. Currently, the only way to "cure" the disease is to identify specific allergies and remove them from the asthmatic's surroundings. This can now be done fairly easily if the asthma is caused by one or two identifiable allergens (e.g., a cat or hamster). However, most of the time, curing the disease is not as simple as this, because there may be many allergens causing the problem or because the asthma may be non-allergic. With the identification of the abnormal gene for asthma, it may be possible eventually to undertake so-called genetic engineering in people with the disease to effect a cure, but such treatments, if possible at all, are probably many decades away.

23 Common Questions About Asthma Answered

Q. Will my child grow out of asthma?

A. Surveys show that about half of children with asthma grow out of it when they are teenagers. The remainder go on to have asthma as adults (and these tend to be the children with the most troublesome asthma). Adults who have asthma do not grow out of it, although there will be times when symptoms are more or less troublesome. This means that adults with asthma often need treatment to control asthma for the rest of their lives.

Q. Can asthma be cured?

A. Unfortunately, there is no cure for asthma. By cure, we mean a treatment that will make asthma go away forever. However, eliminating specific allergens (such as exposure to a cat to which you are allergic, if you have no other allergies) may allow you to discontinue all medications unless you are again exposed to cats! For most asthma such relatively simple solutions are not available but there **are** treatments that can completely control the symptoms of asthma if they are taken properly, and these are discussed throughout the book. These treatments, particularly inhaled steroids, are very effective and allow many asthmatics to live symptom-free lives, but as soon as the treatments are stopped, the asthma symptoms come back. This indicates that these drugs suppress inflammation underlying the asthma but do not cure it.

Q. Will exercise help?

A. Exercise is one of the triggers that can bring on asthma, as discussed in *Chapter 8*, and this may discourage people with asthma from taking part in sports activities. However, proper treatment will allow most asthmatics, both children and adults, to exercise normally. Exercise is beneficial for everyone, and the asthmatic should aim to keep as fit as possible. In the past, there was interest in the idea that exercise itself helped asthma, but there is no evidence that exercise specifically benefits asthma.

Q. Do breathing exercises help?

A. Breathing exercises are special ways of breathing in and out slowly, with the idea that this will "strengthen the lungs." There is no convincing evidence that breathing exercises specifically help asthma, although learning how to control your breathing so that you don't panic may be useful during acute attacks.

Q. Should I try an ionizer?

A. There are several ionizers on the market that are claimed to help asthma. These machines are meant to create negatively-charged particles (ions), but there is no evidence whatsoever either that negative ions are useful for treating asthma or that ionizers are helpful. Since these machines are expensive, we cannot recommend their use in asthma under any circumstances.

Q. Should I go on a special diet?

A. This is a difficult question to answer, because very little is known about the influence of diet on asthma. Certain foods seem to cause a worsening of asthma symptoms in some people. For example, some people may develop wheezing after eating shellfish, nuts, or strawberries, and this may be associated with severe swelling and tingling of the lips and tongue or an itchy skin rash. This is part of a generalized allergic reaction (anaphylaxis) which could be life threatening. Thus, these foods must be avoided at all cost. In other people, the link between certain foods and asthma is not as obvious. Some common foods (such as potatoes, dairy products, or eggs) may cause worsening of asthma in some people, but the link is difficult to establish because these foods are not easy to avoid and the asthma may not worsen until several hours after eating the suspected food. If you think that your asthma is worse after eating a certain type of food, try avoiding it for several weeks, and see whether this helps your asthma.

For common foods, like dairy products (milk, butter, cream), it is difficult to work out a diet that completely eliminates this type of food. Other asthmatics may experience worsening of symptoms because of **additives** in food. The most common troublesome additive is metabisulphite, which is used as a preservative in certain drinks (including beer and wine), and may be used to wash vegetables, such as lettuce in restaurants. Symptoms usually develop immediately after eating the metabisulphite, so it is normally easy to establish a link. The best policy is avoidance. There are certain strange diets that asthmatics may be recommended, but usually there is no scientific basis for their use (see *Chapter 20*).

Q. Does eating natural food or health food help?

A. There is no reason to suppose that eating organically grown vegetables or health food is of particular benefit in asthma, although these foods are less likely to contain additives like metabisulphite. There is no evidence that chemical fertilizers used in the growing of fruit and vegetables cause problems in asthma.

Q. Are there any precautions to take when going on holidays?

A. The most important thing is to take adequate supplies of your asthma treatment, including any treatment you would normally use for severe attacks (such as a course of steroid tablets). This is particularly important when you go to another country, because the same treatments may not be available there. You should **always** take a list of your treatments (preferably with the generic name of the drug rather than the trade name, since these differ between countries — see *Chapters 10 and 11*). It is safe to have the normal vaccinations (injections) that are needed for some countries (e.g., typhoid and cholera vaccines) and to take antimalaria tablets as these will not worsen asthma. It is also perfectly safe to fly in a pressurized aircraft. Again, make sure you always take your treatment with you since airplanes rarely have any emergency treatments for asthma attacks on board.

Q. Will I pass asthma on to my children?

A. You may pass asthma on to your children although asthma often develops in children with no family history whatever. Asthma and other allergic diseases such as rhinitis ("hay fever") tend to run in families, so that children with a strong family history of allergic disorders are more likely to get it. However, even if both parents have allergies or asthma, we do not know if their children will develop these problems. Indeed if there are several children in the family, some may get allergies or asthma and some may not. Furthermore, some children in the family may develop it more severely than others. Fortunately, today most asthma can be well controlled, so that it is rarely the problem it once was. You can expect your child with asthma to lead a completely normal life as long as the correct medications are taken in adequate doses under the supervision of knowledgeable doctors.

Q. Is asthma all in the mind?

A. Asthma is **never** "all in the mind." Asthma is an inflammatory condition of the airways caused by certain allergic factors (allergens) in the environment, chemicals in the workplace, or of unknown cause (probably started by a viral illness). Nevertheless, most asthmatics notice that their asthma tends to be worse when they are under considerable emotional stress. Life is made up of many stresses, so it is not realistic to think that this stress-related component can be eliminated. Fortunately, with currently available treatment, the asthma, in the vast majority of people with the disease, can be so well controlled that even major stressful episodes (such as the death of a close relative, breakup with a boyfriend, divorce, or a loss of a job) should have little, if any effect. The key to caring for your asthma is keeping the condition under control at all times by regularly taking medication, even at times when you feel completely well.

Q. Should children go to special asthma classes, camps, or attend a special school?

A. Today, such effective treatment is available for controlling asthma that children should be able to lead a completely normal life and participate in normal activities, just like their non-asthmatic friends. There should be no need for special classes, breathing exercises, asthma camps, or special schools that tend to isolate children and make them feel "different." A child whose asthma is well-controlled with the treatment outlined in *Chapter 11* should be able to engage in almost all sports, undertake virtually any activities, and choose almost any career. (Exceptions to this are obvious). For example, a person who is highly allergic to animals would be wise to avoid occupations that involve intense exposure, such as animal handling in careers such as veterinary medicine and horse training.

Q. Should I move to another house, and would a change of climate help?

A. Changing where you live is unlikely to be helpful in the long term, because if you are an allergic person, you will soon become allergic to various things such as pollens at your new home. Thus, if you live in Canada, there is little point in moving to Arizona, where communities have turned deserts into lush lawns and floral gardens. Similarly, if you live in the United Kingdom, there is no point in emigrating to Australia. On the other hand, if you are allergic to domestic pets or house dust mites, removing these from your environment as much as possible will certainly result in marked improvement in the allergic complaints.

Q. Should I get rid of my pets?

A. If your pet cat, dog, hamster, bird, etc. is the cause of your asthma or "hay fever," you would be wise to eliminate the cause of your problems from your environment. Just because you have asthma or "hay fever" does not mean that your pet is at fault, and you should discuss this question in detail with your doctor. Skin tests to determine whether your pet might be causing the problem may be helpful in making this decision, but you should remember that about one person in four with no allergic complaints may have a positive skin test anyway. The best way of finding out if you should get rid of your pet is to remove the pet from the house from about 3 months, do a thorough house cleaning, and see if your complaints and your treatment needs (especially a decrease in bronchodilator [reliever] puffs) greatly improve during the time the pet is away. If they do, it is likely that the pet is at fault, and you could actually confirm this by again exposing yourself to the pet for a short time to see if the symptoms come back. If you do the latter, you should do it cautiously and for a relatively short time, and you should be ready to treat yourself with a bronchodilator (reliever) inhaler if you become breathless or wheezy.

Q. Could I die of an asthma attack?

A. You could die of an asthma attack, and occasionally people with asthma do die. However, to die of asthma is extremely rare and almost never occurs if the asthma is properly treated. The proper treatment is outlined in great detail in *Chapter 11* and stresses the fact that you must keep the asthma under good control by using medications that suppress the inflammation that is at the root of the asthmatic condition. Those people that die of asthma (with the exception of the extremely rare person that reacts dramatically to things such as nuts or shellfish) are the ones who do not keep their asthma under good control. When the asthma goes out of control, they do not start their cortisone tablets soon enough or in large enough doses. Before asthma becomes life-threatening, it has usually been deteriorating for many days. It is during that time that awareness of deterioration should lead to effective treatment with larger doses of the inhaled medications that you are taking, or if those do not work fairly quickly, starting prednisolone pills in large doses (see the action plan in *Chapter 11* and on your asthma card). If the prednisolone pills do not produce improvement within 3 or 4 hours or if you are getting worse quickly, you should go to the nearest hospital emergency department **at once**. Nowadays, deaths from asthma are largely unnecessary.

Q. Should I have the influenza vaccine?

A. Yes. You should have the influenza vaccine before the beginning of each 'flu season. This is because viruses change, and last year's vaccination will not do any good for this year's flu. People with asthma are at high risk of serious flare-ups during viral illnesses, and so you should have the flu vaccine to avoid serious viral infections of your nose and lungs.

Q. Will asthma give me lung cancer?

A. No. There is absolutely no connection between asthma and lung cancer. Cigarette smoking is the main cause of lung cancer and asthmatics should never smoke.

Q. Will asthma cause permanent damage to my lungs, such as emphysema?

A. Asthma may cause chronic changes in your lungs similar to emphysema after you have had it for a long time, but this occurs mainly if it is poorly treated or if you smoke! You can help to avoid permanent injury to your lungs by keeping the asthma well controlled at all times and by immediately and vigorously treating asthma flare-ups. If you **smoke tobacco** or **anything else**, you should stop at once.

Q. Will asthma have a harmful effect on my heart or lead to heart attacks?

A. No. Asthma will not affect your heart if it is well controlled. However, if asthma is poorly treated or if you smoke, you may damage your heart. Severe asthma attacks leading to low levels of oxygen in your blood may cause heart problems or may rarely even help to cause a heart attack. So, keep your asthma under good control and **Don't smoke!**

Q. Will asthma medicines injure my heart?

A. It is unlikely that, if used properly, asthma medicines will damage your heart. The aerosol medicines are especially safe, although some doctors have claimed that these sprays may be harmful and even cause death. This is not true as long as you follow your doctor's instructions and stop using additional puffs if you develop marked trembling, a pounding or irregular heartbeat, or chest pain and tightness. If such side effects occur you should contact a doctor at once.

Q. Can people with asthma travel by airplane?

A. Yes, as long as the asthma is under control and you have your bronchodilator (reliever) inhaler and prednisolone medicines with you (not in the checked luggage), so that you can use these if necessary.

Q. Will pregnancy make my asthma worse?

A. If the asthma was well controlled before the pregnancy, it will probably go on being well controlled with the same medication during the pregnancy and after the baby is delivered. Some pregnant women with asthma need much less medication during pregnancy, but some need more to keep the asthma under control. Fortunately, the inhaled asthma medicines used to control asthma and the prednisolone tablets used **only** to treat occasional flare-ups **will not harm the baby**.

Q. Will asthma medicines harm my baby during pregnancy or by getting into the breast milk.

A. No, not if you use aerosol medicines, especially if you use the metered dose inhaler with an add-on device that greatly reduces the amount of medication deposited in the throat.

Q. Can I become "addicted" to my asthma inhalers?

A. No. Using asthma inhalers regularly to control the disease does not make you "dependent" on them. Asthma is caused by inflammation of the air passages which in turn causes spasm of the airways, swelling of the lining and excessive secretions. Taking your preventer medicines regularly in adequate doses should control the inflammation, making it much less necessary to use bronchodilators (relievers).

Q. If I use my inhalers regularly perhaps they won't work when I need them.

A. On the contrary, if you use the antiinflammatory (preventer) medicines such as inhaled steroids regularly your asthma will become well controlled and you may, with time, need less preventer aerosol and many less bronchodilator (reliever) puffs.

145

Appendix

FOODS CONTAINING YELLOW DYE (TARTRAZINE)

Tartrazine is a food colouring (FD + C.5) that gives foods and some drug tablets an "appealing" bright yellow appearance. Examples of foods that contain tartrazine include the following:

Carbohydrates	Fats	Proteins
Some sweet baked goods	Butter	Prepared meats
Sweets	Coloured margarine	
Breakfast cereals	Coloured dairy products (cheese,	
Gelatine (e.g., jelly dessert)	butter, yogurt)	
Potato and other chips		
Cheesies		
Canned fruits		
Ice cream colouring		
Cough lozenges		
Mustard		
Prepackaged gravy		
Toothpaste		

FOODS CONTAINING SALICYLATE

Acetylsalicylic acid (ASA) or aspirin, as it is commonly known, is part of many over-the-counter and prescribed medications. Asthmatics, especially those with known ASA (or other NSAID, *see Chapter 8*) sensitivity **must** avoid these drugs or compound medicines containing them.

ASA is also used as a food preservative, and it may occur naturally in foods in lower concentrations, where it is not as great a problem. **However, avoid ASA wherever possible**. Examples of foods that contain ASA include the following:

Carbohydrates	Fats	Proteins
Alcoholic beverages	Ice cream	Hot dogs
Ciders	Sandwich spreads	Cooked meats
Soft drinks/sodas	Chocolate	
Chewing gum	Pasteurized cheese	
All vegetables except pickles, tomatoes, cucumber	Margarine	
Raisin or other sweet bread		
Cold/hot cereals except puffed rice and wheat		
Cake mix/manufactured cookies/cakes		
All juices except pineapple, pear, grapefruit, cranberry		
Many fruits/berries (e.g., apples, peaches, plums, cherries, apricots, grapes, raisins, oranges, strawberries, raspberries)		
Cloves		
Licorice		
Toothpaste		

FOODS CONTAINING METABISULPHITE

Metabisulphite is a food preservative that is added to many fresh, pickled, and processed foods. It is also added to most beer and wine (scrutinize all labels carefully). Examples of foods that contain metabisulphites include the following:

Carbohydrates	Fats	Proteins
Vinegar	Cheeses	Sausages
Beer		
Wine		
Apple and other fruit cider or juices		
Gelatine (e.g., jelly)		
Dill and other pickles		
Potatoes		
Dried vegetables		

DUST CONTROL FOR ALLERGY TO THE HOUSE DUST MITE

Dust can trigger symptoms in many people because it irritates the sensitive linings of the eyes, nose, or bronchial tubes. It can trigger symptoms in some people because they are allergic to it. In both situations, it is useful to reduce your exposure to dust. This can be reasonably accomplished in the following ways:

1. Use a damp or oiled cloth or mop when dusting. This collects the dust rather than scatters it.

2. Vacuum carpets thoroughly and frequently. When possible, close the doors to other rooms and open the windows in the room being vacuumed to allow as much dust as possible to escape.

3. Before turning the boiler on for the first time each winter, place a damp cheesecloth over the vents; this filters extra dust.

4. Change or wash your boiler filter monthly.

5. When changing bedding, avoid shaking the sheets.

6. Vacuum the mattress and pillows each time you change the sheets.

7. Use foam or fibre-filled pillows; feathers are allergenic and tend to be dust collectors.

8. Use blankets that can be easily washed in a washing machine and that are made from synthetic fibre, (i.e., acrylic, dacron, or polyester). However, if woollen blankets are used, rinsing the blankets in water containing one tablespoon of linseed oil cuts down the dust by 80 percent and does not make the blanket greasy. Avoid quilts, duvets, or eiderdowns, which collect dust.

9. Avoid old furniture and mattresses stuffed with kapok or horse hair.

10. Keep laundry and boiler rooms clean and well vacuumed. Vent driers to the outside.

11. Do not over humidify in winter.

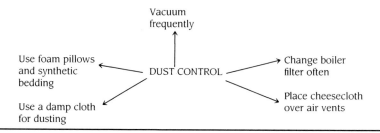

147

AVOIDING ATMOSPHERIC POLLEN AND MOULD SPORES IF YOU ARE ALLERGIC TO THEM

If you are allergic to the following:

(,) tree pollen occurring between mid-April and early June

(,) grass pollen occurring between early May and the end of July

(,) Mould spores occurring throughout the summer and autumn, especially between July and October

You can reduce your exposure to these particles in season in the following ways:

1. Keep windows and doors closed to prevent the particles from entering the home. An air-conditioner will help you to do this in hot weather.

2. Avoid being outside when the counts are highest, i.e., on sunny days in the morning and afternoon. The counts are lowest immediately after rain, in the evening and at night.

3. Avoid situations of high exposure. Exposure to pollen and mould spores is increased by cutting grass, camping, and going into barns. Exposure to mould spores is also increased by sweeping up leaves and working with compost heaps.

4. If you take a holiday, go out of season or go to an area with low counts.

5. If you use a humidifier, add an anti-mould solution to the water (available in hardware stores and chemists).

AVOIDING ANIMALS AND BIRDS IF YOU ARE ALLERGIC TO THEM

Allergy to animals and birds usually causes more trouble in winter months because the house is closed up, the pet is indoors more, and you are also indoors more.

If there is allergy to a pet:

1. It should be removed from the home.

2. If you are not willing to remove the pet (and this may be reasonable if symptoms have not been too troublesome), you can reduce exposure in all of the following ways:

   a) by keeping the pet outdoors as much as possible.

   b) by not allowing the pet in the bedroom.

   c) by only allowing the pet to enter certain rooms, and by keeping the pet off furniture, which tends to collect allergens.

   d) by having the pet washed and brushed frequently by someone else.

   e) by having another family member feed and care for the pet, remembering that clothes worn by that person will have allergens on them.

3. Remember that there are medicines that can be taken to relieve or prevent symptoms of asthma, rhinitis, or conjunctivitis. These may be useful when you do not keep a pet yourself, but will be exposed to one when visiting the home of friends. In this situation, also ask if the pet can be kept out of the room that you are in while you are there.

The extent to which a pet is making your symptoms worse can be tested by a trial period of 3 or 4 months, during which the pet is removed from the home (and the home is thoroughly cleaned and ventilated) or during which you are away from home.

EXERCISE!

Exercise is beneficial for everyone. If you are fit, you will be able to do more work. For example, you will be able to climb a flight of stairs easier than someone who is unfit. People with chest disease often avoid exercise, but exercise is beneficial to them. Exercise strengthens the heart and body muscles, makes better use of oxygen and generally improves the sense of well-being.

If you are short of breath when you exercise, the following are some points to keep in mind:

1. Each person is capable of different amounts of exercise depending on the severity of the problem.

2. Daily activities around the house do not provide enough exercise. You need something more strenuous and continuous.

3. Start with easy activities such as walking on a level for 10 minutes twice a day, and increase to 30 minutes. Then add more strenuous activities such as walking uphill, cycling, or jogging.

4. Exercise should be done every day. It does not have to be exhausting in order to improve fitness. In fact, regular exercise such as walking is more beneficial than occasional stressful exercise like running. A brisk walk of 3 kilometres (2 miles) daily will keep you reasonably fit. This should not take more than 15 to 30 minutes.

5. Exercise indoors when it is cold or damp and when air pollution counts are high, if these factors bother you. A stationary bicycle or stair stepping provide good indoor exercise.

6. If exercise brings on shortness of breath, use an inhaled bronchodilator 5 to 10 minutes before you start.

GLOSSARY OF TERMS

Accessory (add-on) devices Tubes or containers varying in size and volume, often with a valve into which aerosol medication can be sprayed from a pressurized canister metered dose inhaler and from which the aerosol can be reliably inhaled. In addition to assuring aerosol delivery and increasing the benefits of aerosol treatment, these devices also reduce side effects.

Adrenaline A natural body hormone that increases the heart rate, constricts blood vessels so that an individual looks pale, and opens up air passages. It is used to treat anaphylaxis and in the past was used commonly to treat asthma and other allergic reactions.

Aerosol A fine mist of medication that is the best way to treat diseases of the airways such as asthma.

Allergen A substance that causes a particular kind of inflammation as a result of an allergic reaction. Examples are allergy to cats, ragweed pollen (hay fever), and foods (shellfish, peanut butter).

Anaphylaxis A severe and life-threatening allergic reaction that may cause blood pressure to drop, resulting in shock. There is also swelling of the air passages so that breathing is almost impossible. Such reactions must be treated quickly with adrenaline, or death may result.

Antibiotic A medication used to treat infections.

Beta-agonist A type of medication used to relieve asthma attacks rapidly but temporarily. Ventolin, Berotec, Bricanyl, and Pro Air are examples of different kinds of beta-agonists. This group of medications provides short-lived relief of symptoms but does not treat the underlying inflammation. While these medications can be taken in tablet or liquid form or by injection, the best way to use them is by means of an aerosol spray.

Beta-blockers A group of medications usually used to treat high blood pressure or heart disease. These oppose the effect of the body's natural beta-agonists or beta-agonist medications. Beta-blockers must almost never be used in patients with asthma because they could cause severe airway constriction, leading to life-threatening asthma or even death. Fortunately, many other kinds of medications are available to treat the conditions often treated with beta-blockers.

Bronchi These are the air passages that extend from the voice box to the air sacs in the lung. The bronchi become seriously narrowed in asthma because of inflammation, which causes swelling of their walls, constriction of the smooth muscle within the walls, and plugging with secretions produced by the mucous glands in their walls.

Bronchoconstriction The narrowing of the airways that occurs when the smooth muscle in their walls contracts in response to irritation caused by such things as cold air, fog, or tobacco smoke or as a result of inhaling an allergen to which sensitization has occurred.

Bronchodilator This is a drug that opens airways by relaxing the muscle in their walls. If most of the narrowing is caused by inflammatory swelling, bronchodilators may not work very effectively; this is usually the case if the asthma is not well controlled. If the asthma is well controlled, bronchodilators should be needed only rarely. These medications are best taken by inhalation but are also available as tablets or liquids, and for injection.

Cardiac "asthma" A term used by doctors to describe the wheezing that sometimes accompanies heart failure. It is important that this not be confused with asthma because the treatment is completely different.

Congestive heart failure A disease in which, because the heart has been damaged, fluid accumulates in the lungs. This may cause wheezing and mislead doctors into thinking that asthma is the problem.

Corticosteroids Corticosteroids, or steroids as they are often called, are one of an important group of natural hormones found in the body. They have a powerful effect in reducing inflammation and are thus used to keep asthma under control. Steroids are also used in larger doses to bring asthma under control when it deteriorates or after an attack of asthma has occurred. The steroids used to treat asthma are not the same medications that have been in the news lately because they were used illegally by athletes to build muscles. These medications can be taken by inhalation, as tablets, intravenously, or by injection into muscles. The best and safest way to use corticosteroids is by inhalation because this greatly decreases potential side effects. When corticosteroids are inhaled, such minute doses are used that the effects are almost entirely local in the airways. This type of drug is called a "preventer" because, by taking it regularly, the inflammation underlying asthma is prevented and the asthma brought under control.

Cromoglycate (cromolyn) This is also a medication that suppresses inflammation and acts as a "preventer" of inflammation and controller of asthma. It is not a bronchodilator or "reliever" like the beta-agonists. It is taken only by inhalation and may be effective for treating mild to moderate asthma, particularly in children. It has few, if any, side effects.

Eosinophil This is one of the cells most commonly associated with the inflammation of the airways called asthma and with allergic rhinitis. These cells are found in the blood and tissues of patients with these conditions and may actually contribute to the injury and inflammation.

Forced expired volume in one second (FEV$_1$) The volume of air that can be forcibly exhaled in one second after a full breath has been taken. When the airways are narrowed in asthma, much less air can be exhaled in one second (like breathing out through a straw). The predicted reading for any given individual depends on age and height.

Gastro-oesophageal reflux A condition that results from regurgitation of stomach juices into the oesophagus (gullet). This may cause chest pain, heartburn, and cough. If the stomach secretion gets into the back of the throat at night during sleep, a little may trickle into the lungs and cause severe coughing, wheezing, and sometimes pneumonia. Although the chest symptoms of this condition may be similar to asthma, it is important to distinguish the two because the treatments are completely different. Sometimes asthma and reflux occur together; this may make diagnosis difficult.

Histamine A hormone that is produced by certain cells (mast cells) in the body. This hormone regulates certain cell functions and is produced in great excess during allergic reactions. It causes blood vessels to widen and become porous, thus letting fluid leak into the skin (hives) and into the walls of the air passages, causing them to swell. It also causes narrowing of the airways because it makes the smooth muscle in the airway walls constrict. In the nose, this hormone causes congestion and excess secretions. Antihistamine medications may counteract the effects in the skin, eyes, and nose but are rarely helpful in treating asthma.

Infection Infection of the airways usually leads to cough and phlegm and in asthmatics may also cause wheezing, chest tightness, and shortness of breath. Infection is caused by bacteria, viruses, and other microscopic organisms. Infection of the lung tissue is called pneumonia. There are also condtions in which inflammation causes the symptoms.

Inflammation This word describes reactions of the body to injury, with which we all are familiar. The result is redness, swelling, and pain (in the skin) or narrowing and irritability (in the airways). Examples of inflammation are sunburn, boils, ingrown toenails, arthritis, and asthma. Inflam-

mation is the way the body may defend itself against infecting bacteria and viruses, but the result of the battle may sometimes be damage to body tissues. In asthma, inflammation leads to swelling, bronchoconstriction, and the production of excess secretions, all of which may contribute to narrowing of the airways. Similar changes may occur in the nose, skin, or eyes. Inflammation of the air passages may cause mainly cough rather than shortness of breath, wheezing, and chest tightness.

Inhaler A device that provides aerosol medicine from a portable unit. Examples are metered dose inhalers (with a pressurized canister) and powder inhalers.

Mast cells Large cells normally present in the body but increased in asthma and allergic conditions. These cells are full of small packets of hormones such as histamine. These hormones take part in the allergic reaction and act to increase inflammation and cause constriction of the airways by contraction of the airway muscles and by increasing secretions and airway swelling.

Metered dose inhaler (MDI) A device used by many asthmatics to relieve airway narrowing by means of aerosol treatment. The aerosol comes from a small pressurized canister or from a powder inhaler. The medication can be inhaled directly (if coordination is good and there is no concern about side effects) or through an accessory device.

Nebulizer A device that creates a medication mist or aerosol from liquid medications. It requires an external power source (squeeze bulb, air compressor, or ultrasonic electrical unit). Compared to MDIs, these devices are fairly inefficient and expensive to buy and operate.

Peak flow meter A small device for measuring the amount of air that can be blown out of the lungs forcefully. The measurement is called the peak expiratory flow rate (PEFR). This measurement tells how severe the asthma is from one time to another, indicates how well the bronchodilator (reliever) is working, and is sometimes used for doing research on new medications.

Prednisone Prednisolone A form of corticosteroid medicine that is one of the most powerful suppressors of inflammation. It comes in the form of tablets or as an intramuscular or intravenous injection. It is often used to treat severe asthma attacks by means of fairly large doses for one or two weeks at a time and is occasionally needed in very severe asthma for maintenance treatment, almost always along with inhaled steroids and bronchodilators. It is well known that this kind of medication may cause (sometimes serious) side effects when used for many weeks or months. It should therefore be used in the smallest possible doses and for the shortest possible period of time.

When used for up to 2 or 3 weeks, the side effects are rarely a problem and usually disappear quickly when the medication is reduced in dose or stopped. Some patients may be able to take small doses for many years without problems.

Rhinitis Inflammation of the lining of the nasal passages, which leads to swelling, plugging, and sneezing. Excess mucous secretion causes a runny nose.

Secretions Fluid produced by glands in the body called mucous glands. The secretion is often called mucus. Coughing up secretions from the chest always indicates an abnormality in the air passages. The secretions may be clear, yellow, or green. Coloured secretions always indicate inflammation, although not necessarily infection. Asthma that is not well controlled may cause coloured secretions to be coughed up.

Signs Your doctor's findings when he/she examines you. An example is whistling noises heard through a stethoscope during an asthma attack.

Spirometer An instrument for measuring vital capacity (VC) and one second forced expired volume (FEV_1). These measurements are made by blowing into an electronic device or a balloon-like machine.

Stethoscope An instrument your doctor uses to listen to your heart and lungs.

Symptoms The reports or complaints you tell your doctor. Examples are breathlessness, cough, and wheeze.

Theophylline A medication used many years ago for treating asthma. It is taken by mouth or given by intravenous injection. It is a reliever (bronchodilator) type of medication and does not have an effect on the underlying inflammation. This medication causes many side effects and is now used much less commonly.

Vital capacity This refers to the amount of air that can be blown out of the lungs completely after a full breath has been taken.

MEDICAL SUMMARY CARD

Name: Birth date: /   /

Address:

Phone:

In case of emergency contact:

Name:

Address:

Phone:

Nat. Ins No:

Family Doctor: Phone:

Hosp:

USE PENCIL TO ALLOW FOR FUTURE CHANGES

DIAGNOSIS:
ALLERGIES:

OTHER MEDICAL PROBLEMS:

FUNCTION TESTS:	DATE	BEST	USUAL	PRED
Peak Flow				
FEV$_1$				
VC				

MEDICATIONS:	5.
1.	6.
2.	7.
3.	8.
4.	9.

USE PENCIL TO ALLOW FOR FUTURE CHANGES

153

ASTHMA ACTION PLAN

Complete this with your doctor's help. (Use pencil to allow future changes.)

The steroid tablet is _____ mg per tablet.

Your maintenance dose is _____ mg/ _____.

The bronchodilator (reliever) is _____ μg per puff.

Your maintenance dose is _____ puffs _____ x/d as needed.

The anti-inflammatory (preventer) is _____ μg per puff.

Your maintenance dose is _____ puffs _____ x/d regularly.

* Your best peak flow is _____ L/min.

ACTION

Asthma gradually worsening?

Symptoms: more breathlessness, asthma at night, cough, chest tight in AM, using bronchodilator more than _____ x/day
* Peak flow reduced 15% or more to below _____ L/min following bronchodilator for 2 days in a row.

A Remove the cause if possible.
Increase Preventer _____ to _____ puffs _____ x/day. (Usually double the maintenance dose.)

Improving within 24 hours?

YES
Continue **A** for 2 weeks, then resume maintenance treatment.

NO
B Start steroid _____ tabs/day for _____ days
AND CONTACT YOUR DOCTOR.
Then _____ tabs/d for _____ days.

Improving within _____ hours?

YES
Continue **B**, then resume maintenace treatment.

NO
C GET MEDICAL ATTENTION AT ONCE!

Severe Asthma Attack

D Take _____ puffs of bronchodilator (1 every 30 secs) AT ONCE.

Improving within 15 minutes?

YES
START A

NO
E Take _____ additional puff of bronchodilator each minute to max of _____ puffs. Stop if trembly or severe palpitations occur.

Breathlessness improving within 15 minutes?

YES
START B

NO
GET MEDICAL ATTENTION AT ONCE!

* Monitor peak flow on your doctor's advice.

Follow your doctor's advice.

Index

For references to specific medicines please check under Drug, Treatment and generic type